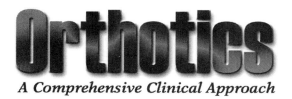

Orthotics

A Comprehensive Clinical Approach

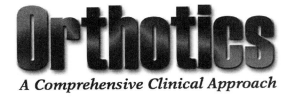

Orthotics
A Comprehensive Clinical Approach

Joan E. Edelstein, MA, PT, FISPO
Program in Physical Therapy
Columbia University
New York, NY

Jan Bruckner, PhD, PT
Department of Physical Therapy
Thomas Jefferson University
Philadelphia, PA

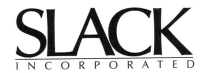

An innovative information, education and management company
6900 Grove Road • Thorofare, NJ 08086

The procedures and practices described in this book should be implemented in a manner consistent with the professional standards set for the circumstances that apply in each specific situation. Every effort has been made to confirm the accuracy of the information presented and to correctly relate generally accepted practices. The authors, editor, and publisher cannot accept responsibility for errors or exclusions or for the outcome of the application of the material presented herein. There is no expressed or implied warranty of this book or information imparted by it.

The work SLACK publishes is peer reviewed. Prior to publication, recognized leaders in the field, educators, and clinicians provide important feedback on the concepts and content that we publish. We welcome feedback on this work.

Printed in the United States of America.

Library of Congress Cataloging-in-Publication Data

Edelstein, Joan E.
    Orthotics : a comprehensive clinical approach / Joan Edelstein, Janice Bruckner.
        p. ; cm.
    Includes bibliographical references and index.
    ISBN 1-55642-416-7 (alk. paper)
    1. Orthopedic apparatus. 2. Prosthesis. I. Bruckner, Jan. II. Title.
    [DNLM: 1. Orthotic Devices. WE 26 E21o 2001]
    RD755 .E345 2001
    617'.9--dc21

                                                                    2001049326

Published by: SLACK Incorporated
                       6900 Grove Road
                       Thorofare, NJ 08086 USA
                       Telephone: 856-848-1000
                       Fax: 856-853-5991
                       www.slackbooks.com

Contact SLACK Incorporated for more information about other books in this field or about the availability of our books from distributors outside the United States.

Authorization to photocopy items for internal or personal use, or the internal or personal use of specific clients, is granted by SLACK Incorporated, provided that the appropriate fee is paid directly to Copyright Clearance Center, 222 Rosewood Drive, Danvers, MA 01923 USA, 978-750-8400. Prior to photocopying items for educational classroom use, please contact the CCC at the address above. Please reference Account Number 9106324 for SLACK Incorporated's Professional Book Division.

For further information on CCC, check CCC Online at the following address: http://www.copyright.com.

Last digit is print number: 10   9   8   7   6   5   4   3   2   1

Contents

ACKNOWLEDGMENTS

We offer profound thanks to Michael Carasik and Haskell Edelstein for their encouragement, comments, and forbearance during our labors on this book. John Bond, Amy Drummond, and Carrie Kotlar of SLACK Incorporated provided unfailingly helpful guidance in bringing the book from dream to reality. Nicole Barbagello assisted with the appendices. Our teachers, patients, and colleagues shape our professional insights, for which we are most grateful. Finally, we acknowledge the contributions of our students, who continually challenge us to harmonize the practical and research aspects of clinical experience.

ABOUT THE AUTHORS

Joan E. Edelstein, MA, PT, FISPO, is a world-renowned authority in orthotics and prosthetics. After graduating from New York University, NY, magna cum laude, she entered clinical practice in the Children's Division of the Institute of Physical Medicine and Rehabilitation, subsequently renamed the Rusk Institute of New York University, where she became chief physical therapist. When invited to join the faculty of the University of Wisconsin, Madison, she began the academic phase of her career. Returning to New York, she became a senior research scientist at New York University's Prosthetics and Orthotics Program, originally part of the College of Engineering, later a division of the Department of Orthopedic Surgery and the School of Education. She conducted laboratory and field-testing of a wide variety of prostheses and orthoses for the upper and lower limbs, as well as trunk orthoses. She is highly regarded for her enthusiastic instruction in the postgraduate courses offered to physicians, therapists, orthotists, prosthetists, pedorthists, and rehabilitation counselors. She pioneered the establishment of the first undergraduate curriculum leading to the baccalaureate in prosthetics and orthotics. Upon the closing of the New York University program, she became an associate professor of clinical physical therapy at the College of Physicians and Surgeons, Columbia University, New York, NY, and is director of the Program in Physical Therapy.

Professional contributions beyond the university include service as a member of the Scientific Merit Review Board of the Department of Veterans Affairs. She has been editor or member of the editorial boards of *Archives of Physical Medicine and Rehabilitation, Journal of the Association of Children's Prosthetic-Orthotic Clinics, Journal of Rehabilitation Research and Development,* and *Physical and Occupational Therapy in Geriatrics.* She was honored by being named a Fellow of the International Society for Prosthetics and Orthotics.

Professor Edelstein conducts courses throughout North America, Europe, Africa, and the Middle East. She has been a keynote speaker at professional conferences and congresses. A prolific contributor to the professional literature, her numerous journal articles, book chapters, monographs, and books pertain to all phases of the field.

Jan Bruckner, PhD, PT, has been a practicing clinician since 1977. She received her bachelor of arts in anthropology cum laude from Barnard College, Columbia University, NY, in 1975 and her masters of science in physical therapy from Sargent College, Boston University, Mass, in 1977. She worked in a Rochester, NY, geriatric facility for 1 year and then joined the US Peace Corps. After serving 2 1/2 years in Barbados practicing geriatrics, pediatrics, and sports medicine, she returned to work for United Cerebral Palsy of New York State in New York City and, later, for Manhattan Developmental Center. These programs served the Willowbrook class clients, and she became familiar with the infamous Willowbrook hepatitis study. In 1982, she joined the faculty of the Indiana University Physical Therapy Program and began her doctoral studies in physical anthropology and bioethics the following year. She earned her masters in bioanthropology in 1992 and her PhD in bioanthropology with a minor in bioethics in 1993. She moved to Boston and joined the physical therapy faculty of Northeastern University in 1993. Since 1998, she has been the Director of Research for the Department of Physical Therapy at Thomas Jefferson University in Philadelphia, Pa.

Dr. Bruckner developed an interest in orthoses while working with clients during her Peace Corps service and during her tenure at United Cerebral Palsy. She took several courses with Ms. Edelstein when Ms. Edelstein was on the faculty of New York University's Orthotics and Prosthetics Program. She has been teaching prosthetics and orthotics to physical therapy students since 1985. Her interest in the subject led her to develop a new ballet shoe that minimizes pain, deformity, and disability in dancers who perform *en pointe.* She received a patent for this design in May 2001.

Dr. Bruckner has been active in numerous professional organizations, including the American Physical Therapy Association and the American Physical Anthropological Association. With her Thomas Jefferson University physical therapy students, Dr. Bruckner runs a foot clinic in Center City Philadelphia for people who are homeless. She has written a book on observational gait analysis; book chapters on bioethics and transfer techniques; and numerous articles on anthropology, bioethics, osteology, and physical therapy care for people who are homeless.

Dr. Bruckner currently lives with her husband, Dr. Michael Carasik, in Center City Philadelphia where both are actively involved in the community. Dr. Bruckner serves as the fund-raising chair of the Center City Eruv Corporation, participates in the Kesher Israel Women's Davening Group, and is a member of the Society Hill Civic Association. Among her hobbies, Dr. Bruckner enjoys gardening, quilting, and refinishing furniture.

PREFACE

Orthoses play an integral part in the rehabilitation of many patients. An infant born with dislocated hips and a centenarian who has sustained a stroke are both likely to wear orthoses. Whether the patient is an athlete coping with a torn medial meniscus or a retired teacher adjusting to drop foot caused by diabetic neuropathy, optimum management involves interaction between a knowledgeable clinician, the patient, and his or her family members. The premise of *Orthotics: A Comprehensive Clinical Approach* is that prescribing and utilizing orthoses is best achieved when the patient is thoroughly evaluated, from biomechanical, neuromusculoskeletal, and psychosocial perspectives. Clinicians should consider the full gamut of orthotic designs and materials to arrive at a prescription with which the patient will comply and benefit.

As clinicians, teachers, and research investigators, we recognize that physical therapists, physicians, occupational therapists, orthotists, pedorthists, rehabilitation nurses, other health care providers, and students in these professions can serve patients best by understanding the interaction of orthoses with patients' neuromuscular, musculoskeletal, cardiopulmonary, and integumentary systems. Often, several orthoses can improve function of a given individual, but the clinical art is to select the one device among the possible choices that has the greatest likelihood of being accepted by the patient.

The breadth of the field of orthotics is reflected in the plan of this book, which is intended as both a text for the student and a reference for the practitioner. The first chapter introduces key concepts of terminology, personnel involved in orthotic management, prescription considerations, biomechanics, and materials and construction methods. Subsequent chapters describe a wide range of orthoses for the lower limb, trunk and neck, and upper limb, as well as specialized information about orthoses for paraplegia and soft tissue disorders. Discussions highlight distinctive features of well-fitting orthoses, advantages, potential drawbacks, and evaluation procedures. The final chapter addresses treatment planning and goal setting. To enhance the value of the book as a reference, appendices include lists of professional organizations; sources of orthoses, materials, and components; and helpful Internet websites.

Thought-provoking questions and case studies at the end of most chapters should foster clinical reasoning and problem-solving skills. Point/Counterpoint sections demonstrate how experienced clinicians might manage the same patient in different ways. By the same token, we are aware of regional differences in patient care, as well as ongoing changes in orthotic design and materials. We assume that the reader understands the biomechanics of normal and pathological gait, as well as anatomical terminology. We hope to inspire broader thinking about clinical management and a deeper understanding of rehabilitation so that patients may achieve the highest level of function and well-being.

Joan E. Edelstein, MA, PT, FISPO
Jan Bruckner, PhD, PT

Chapter 1

Introduction to Orthotics

"Begin at the beginning," the King said gravely, "and go on till you come to the end; then stop."
Lewis Carroll, Alice in Wonderland

The field of orthotics includes appliances for the lower limb, trunk, neck, and upper limb. This chapter outlines key concepts that apply to orthoses, regardless of the body segment on which the device is worn. What is an orthosis? Who is involved with orthotic prescription? How ancient are orthoses? What mechanical principles govern orthotic design? What materials are used in orthoses? How are orthoses constructed?

TERMINOLOGY

Orthosis derives from the Greek expression "making straight." An orthosis is an orthopedic appliance used to support, align, prevent, or correct deformities of a body part or to improve the function of moveable parts of the body.[1] *Orthesis* is sometimes used to denote an orthosis; *brace* is synonymous with orthosis. A *splint* is a temporary orthosis. Some of the other common terms that denote particular orthotic designs include sling, corset, pressure garment, and cuff. *Surgical appliance* is the broad category that includes orthoses. *Orthotic* is the adjective relating to orthoses, but it is sometimes used to designate a foot orthosis. An *orthotist* is the healthcare practitioner who designs, fabricates, and fits patients with orthoses. *Orthotics* refers to the field of knowledge relating to orthoses and their use.

HISTORICAL BACKGROUND

To understand the evolution of contemporary orthoses and to appreciate differences in orthotic practice, it is useful to highlight the history of orthoses. Additionally, some current orthoses are known by the name of the developer.

Paintings from the fifth Egyptian dynasty, 2750 to 2625 BCE (Before Common Era) depict men wearing orthoses. Various braces and splints for the treatment of fractures, dislocations, and congenital deformities have been attributed to Hippocrates, the Greek physician of the 4th century BCE. Galen, who subscribed to hippocratic teachings, wrote about scoliosis orthoses in the 2nd century CE (Common Era). Ambroise Paré, the "father of modern surgery," who first published his works in 1575, made a perforated steel orthosis for the correction of scoliosis and an ankle-foot orthosis to correct club foot, among many other orthoses and prostheses. Hieronymus Fabricius of Hilden, Germany described in 1607 an orthosis to reduce contractures caused by burns. Nicholas Andry, professor of medicine at the University of Paris, wrote in 1740 about correction and prevention of deformities in children, including trunk orthoses. He coined the word "orthopedic," meaning straight child. Antonio Scarpa, a Venetian surgeon, published an 1803 treatise on congenital foot deformities illustrating several club foot orthoses. The English orthopedist Hugh Owen Thomas designed lower-limb orthoses for weight-bearing, which appeared in his 1875 publication. His contemporary, James Knight, an American surgeon, designed a lumbosacral orthosis that bears his name. The German technician Friederich von Hessing advanced the art of brace-making in the latter part of the 19th century.[2]

PERSONNEL

While historic practice often involved one person's judgment, best practice today usually reflects the considered decision of an orthotic clinic team. Professional members of the team include the orthotist, physician, and physical therapist. Often a pedorthist, occupational therapist, social worker, and other health care professionals, such as a podiatrist, participate in the team. The patient is a key member of the team who contributes important information regarding past orthotic experiences, esthetic preferences, and functional requirements.

Orthotists

In current practice, orthotists have various types of formal preparation, all of which entitle the individual to add the initials CO (Certified Orthotist) or CPO (Certified Prosthetist-Orthotist) to one's name. Orthotists who have been in practice for many years usually have taken a series of brief university courses in various aspects of the field. Newer practitioners are college graduates who have majored in orthotics or in prosthetics and orthotics, or who have completed postgraduate certificate courses. All candidates for certification must complete 1900 hours of supervised clinical experience. An orthotist who passes the certifying examination administered by the American Board for Certification in Orthotics and Prosthetics, Inc. is designated a Certified Orthotist (CO). Some practitioners have completed additional education and examinations and are designated as Certified Prosthetist-Orthotists (CPO). Orthotists who are certified by the Board for Orthotist-Prosthetist Certification add BOC (Board for Orthotist-Prosthetist Certification) to their names. Several states license orthotists.

Pedorthists

Pedorthists specialize in the design, construction, and fitting of foot orthoses, including shoes intended for therapeutic purposes and their modifications. The Board for Certification in Pedorthics examines and certifies pedorthists, who are designated as C.Ped.

Physicians

Physicians, most often specialists in orthopedics or rehabilitation medicine, are responsible for authorizing the orthotic prescription. Board examinations in both specialties include questions pertaining to orthotics. Insurance coverage, which underwrites the cost of most orthoses, ordinarily requires a physician's approval. In principle, any physician can write an orthotic prescription. Nevertheless, the patient is best served when the physician is knowledgeable about contemporary designs and materials. The physician evaluates physical and other personal factors to determine if the patient's disorder may be ameliorated by an orthosis.

Physical Therapists

Part of basic professional education is instruction in the principles governing orthotics and the most frequently prescribed devices as required by the Commission on Accreditation of Physical Therapy Education. Clinical internships usually include interactions with patients who wear orthoses, especially in training them to function with the devices. Questions on orthotic management appear on the licensure examination. Physical therapists have the major responsibility of evaluating the patient's balance, joint excursions, motor power, skin condition, and current and potential function, as well as teaching the patient how to don and doff the orthosis, use it correctly, and maintain it.

Occupational Therapists

Occupational therapists may contribute to orthotic prescription, particularly with regard to patients requiring upper-limb devices. Occupational therapy education includes instruction in the construction of splints and similar appliances. Fieldwork relevant to physical disabilities usually encompasses patients who use orthoses. The National Board for Certification in Occupational Therapy administers an examination that includes questions pertaining to orthotics. The examination is essential both for states licensing occupational therapists and for those that have registration, certification, or trademark laws.

Social Workers and Psychologists

When the patient has psychosocial issues that may affect orthotic prescription or use, the advice of a social worker or psychologist can be helpful. For example, the individual who sustained paraplegia following spinal cord injury may be profoundly depressed and may refuse to participate in a gait-training program that involves wearing an orthosis. A patient with low back pain may decline to relinquish the spinal orthosis, even when it is no longer needed, because the appliance is physical evidence of a sick role that the individual wants to maintain. Counseling can provide psychological support for such people and their families. Social workers may assist with locating sources of funding for orthotic services.

FACTORS IN PRESCRIPTION

Determining the most appropriate orthosis for a given patient at a particular point in the individual's treatment should take into account many considerations. These include the person's present status as evaluated by the various members of the clinic team, the anticipated duration of orthotic use, and the patient's environment, financial resources, and psychosocial concerns.

Clinic Team

The central purpose of the clinic team is to formulate a prescription for an orthosis, evaluate its fit, and assess the wearer's function while wearing it. The larger objective is to manage the patient's rehabilitation, which usually encompasses training with the orthosis and may include the services of a surgeon, rehabilitation nurse, recreation therapist, and other clinicians. In the best of circumstances, the clinic team meets on a regular basis to review candidates for orthoses. Prior to the meeting, the members of the team should have evaluated the patient so that those pertinent findings can be shared with the entire group. As each patient is presented, team members provide key information that may affect prescription, then consider the array of possible designs and materials. The final prescription should represent the considered judgment of the entire team. The team also meets when the orthosis is delivered to ascertain whether it fits and functions properly and also just before the patient is to be discharged to determine if any last-minute adjustments are required. Other team meetings may involve review of the patient's status, with consideration for changing or eliminating the orthosis.

Selection of the most appropriate orthosis for a given individual is a major responsibility. Most patients can manage—to a greater or lesser extent—with a variety of devices. Rarely are components contraindicated. Rather, the clinical challenge is to exercise optimal judgment, taking into account biomechanical requirements of the individual and the many factors that influence acceptance of the orthosis. Ideally, prescription is a shared endeavor by the patient and the professional staff most closely associated with orthotic use.

Prescription Goals

A reasonable starting point for prescription is when the clinic team establishes rational goals for orthotic use. The team may need to set priorities for the patient who has multiple needs. For example, a person with hemiplegia needs to stand to prevent contractures and disuse osteoporosis, to transfer from bed to chair, and to move safely in the community. Although an orthosis may aid the patient in maintaining a stable standing position and transfer from bed to chair, it will not lift the person from a chair or eliminate crevices in the sidewalk, which may interfere with the patient's travels.

Physical Examination

Examination and evaluation should identify the pathomechanical disorders that disturb the individual's function. Abnormal skeletal and articular alignment can interfere with the patient's stability. Muscular weakness places undue stress on joint capsules and compromises the individual's gait. Neuropathies can also hinder walking. The evaluation should include assessment of coordination, sensation, and reflexes. Essential for prescription is an examination of the condition of the skin and subcutaneous tissue. Scar tissue, unhealed wounds, edema, and atrophied areas affect orthotic selection. Another physical factor is vision. Patients with severe impairment need a type of fastening and orthotic design that will give them the best chance of being able to independently don orthoses. Regardless of the body area being considered for an orthosis, the examination should include consideration of the person's hand function. Will the patient be able to manipulate closures on the orthosis or is modification required?

Duration

The patient should be told the duration of orthotic use, both from the point of view of periods during the day when the device is to be worn and with regard to the time of reevaluation of the orthosis weeks or months later. If the orthosis is intended for long-term use, sturdier materials and components are essential.

Places of Use

Orthotic prescription should reflect the places in which the patient is most likely to use the orthosis. Is the person's home spacious enough to permit the individual to engage in an orthotically assisted gait program? A crowded apartment, for example, offers little opportunity for practicing ambulation. In school, the child's primary activity is sitting with relatively brief periods available for standing and walking. In the work environment, the employee may find it expedient to remain in a wheelchair.

Finances

The one potential contraindication to every prescription option is insufficient funds. Either the prescription must be altered to keep within fiscal constraints or adequate funding must be obtained. Social service agencies play a critical role in this regard.

Psychosocial Issues

Although an orthosis may be viewed as a device supporting a body segment, the individual's cognitive, emotional, and social status are critical factors in selecting an orthosis that the patient will accept.

Cognitive Abilities

The clinic team should consider the patient's cognitive abilities, particularly the person's ability to understand donning, using, and maintaining the orthosis. A patient who sustained a cerebrovascular accident, for example, may demonstrate motor apraxia, which can interfere with fitting the paretic arm into a sling.

Orthotic Experience

An imperative component of prescription is the patient's orthotic experience. If the patient has previously worn an orthosis, what features were acceptable? What aspects of design, material, and appearance were disliked? How well did the person function with previous orthoses?

Probable Compliance

The team must estimate the extent of the patient's compliance with the proposed orthotic wear schedule. If the individual expresses unrealistic hopes for spontaneous recovery, then cooperation with a program incorporating orthotic use is doubtful. Conversely, some people do not understand the importance of frequent doffing of the orthosis when it is first delivered in order to check the condition of the skin and other soft tissues. Others overexert themselves in a misguided attempt to accelerate recovery. The rebellious adolescent who refuses to wear a scoliosis orthosis, fearing the ridicule of schoolmates, may be better served by operative management or other intervention. Similarly, the patient who does not or cannot understand the importance of wearing shoes of appropriate design will benefit more from a lower-limb orthosis that is riveted to a suitable shoe. The young adult with spinal cord injury who harbors fantasies regarding the return of function may view wrist-hand orthoses as superfluous.

The conscientious team always considers the patient's preferences. People may view the orthosis as a stigma, identifying the wearer as inadequate or incompetent. If the orthosis is to be worn in school or at work, its appearance is a major issue. Will the patient be embarrassed by the appearance of the orthosis? Ordinarily, the more inconspicuous the orthosis, the better. On the other hand, some patients, such as those with athletic injuries, may express the desire to have an appliance that is brightly colored to highlight their encounters with danger or match their exercise clothes. Children may favor pictures of cartoon characters imbedded in the shells of the orthosis. If the orthosis will be used only at night or in a clinical environment, appearance is less important.

ORTHOTIC NOMENCLATURE

Historically, orthoses were often named for the designer (eg, Thomas ring), the place of origin (eg, Milwaukee brace), or impairment (eg, wrist drop splint). Currently, most orthoses have a generic designation that identifies the involved body part and the orthotic function, although some traditional names remain in common use. For example, many scoliosis orthoses can be described as thoracolumbosacral orthoses. Without a particular designation, such as Boston or Charleston orthosis, one would not know what design was meant.

Lower-Limb Orthoses

Foot orthoses (FOs) may be an insert worn inside the shoe, an internal modification glued inside the shoe, or an external modification secured to the shoe sole or heel. An ankle-foot orthosis (AFO) covers some portion of the foot and leg. The term AFO may be modified to indicate a specific ankle-foot orthosis. For example, an AFO-SA is an ankle-foot orthosis that includes a solid ankle. Knee orthoses (KOs) extend from the distal thigh to the proximal leg. A knee-ankle-foot orthosis (KAFO) encompasses the thigh, leg, and foot. Hip orthoses (HOs) surround the hip. A hip-knee-ankle-foot orthosis (HKAFO) originates on the pelvis and terminates at the foot. A trunk-hip-knee-ankle-foot orthosis (THKAFO) encircles the torso, both thighs and legs, and ends at the feet.

Trunk and Cervical Orthoses

Most trunk orthoses are named for the section of the torso encircled as well as the type of control that the orthosis provides. For example, a lumbosacral flexion-extension control orthosis (LS FEO) extends from the midthoracic area to the inferior pelvis and has vertical bars and a canvas front that restrict the wearer's range of trunk flexion and extension. The current terminology is not entirely consistent (eg, "T" refers to trunk in the context of a lower-limb orthosis but means thoracic if a trunk orthosis is described). Likewise, cervical orthoses are seldom referred to as CO because this also designates a Certified Orthotist. Consequently, names describing the specific orthoses are preferable. Chapter 7 details the full nomenclature for trunk and cervical orthoses.

Upper-Limb Orthoses

Terms used to designate devices for the upper limb follow a similar pattern. SO is a shoulder orthosis, EO is an elbow orthosis, and WHO refers to a wrist-hand orthosis. Because hand and finger orthoses may serve multiple functions, the nomenclature for these appliances is more varied. Chapter 8 provides the major descriptors for upper-limb devices.

BIOMECHANICAL PRINCIPLES

All orthoses apply forces to the body. The therapeutic benefit of the force application may be to resist or assist motion, transfer force, or protect a body part. The amount of force and the area of the body subjected to the force influence the comfort of the orthosis.

Therapeutic Benefits of Orthoses

Resist Motion

Orthoses are used to control excessive or unwanted motion (eg, to prevent a thoracic scoliosis from increasing by strategically placed pads in a trunk orthosis). A woman who has quadriceps paralysis may wear a KAFO that has a mechanical lock to stabilize the knee. A man who sustained spinal cord injury may be fitted with a THKAFO that supports him, immobilizing the hips, knees, and ankles so he can stand. In addition to resisting motion, orthoses can maintain a particular alignment. A hip orthosis can keep the femoral head in the acetabulum for a youngster with Legg-Calvé-Perthes disease. A wrist-hand orthosis can minimize ulnar deviation in a patient with rheumatoid arthritis.

Assist Motion

Orthoses can provide mechanical assistance of weak or paralyzed muscles to enable the wearer to perform a specific function (eg, a wrist-hand orthosis [WHO] may link wrist extension to flex the fingers in a paralyzed hand). A man who sustained laceration of the peroneal nerve is likely to drag his foot during the swing phase of gait, risking a tripping accident. An orthosis that has a plastic or metal spring in the vicinity of the ankle will compensate for the impairment by assisting foot dorsiflexion during the swing phase.

Transfer Force

Orthoses can be designed to transfer forces from one portion of the body to another (eg, a foot orthosis that shifts load from a heel spur to the forefoot). Load transfer is often used in FOs. A woman with metatarsalgia will be more comfortable with a FO that includes a pad underneath the metatarsal shafts. The pad transfers force from the painful metatarsal heads to the less sensitive shafts. An orthosis that incorporates an ischial seat and a patten bottom transfers weight-bearing stress from the pelvis to the distal end of the orthosis, bypassing the skeleton of the lower limb.

Protect Body Parts

Some orthoses protect body areas, preventing deformity or injury. For example, patients with burns need to shield newly grafted skin from secondary trauma. Similarly, the individual with an insensitive and unstable ankle secondary to neuropathic disease will be more stable with a protective AFO.

Comfort

Regardless of its purpose, the orthosis must be comfortable; otherwise, the patient is unlikely to wear it. If an uncomfortable orthosis is worn, it may irritate or injure the skin and underlying structures. A major element in ensuring comfort is minimizing pressure by maximizing the area covered by the orthosis. Another way to improve comfort is to provide sufficient leverage through which the longitudinal segments of the orthosis apply force.

Maximizing Area

The greater the portion of the body that the orthosis covers, the lower the unit pressure. For example, the plastic shell of an AFO, which contacts the entire posterior portion of the leg, is likely to be more comfortable than an upholstered metal calf band of an AFO, which contacts only a 5 cm strip on the proximal leg. Covering a large portion of the body, however, may be uncomfortable because the skin under the orthosis cannot dissipate heat readily. Consequently, the patient should wear a cotton garment under the orthosis because perspiration that accumulates beneath the orthosis can lead to skin maceration. The amount of subcutaneous fat and muscle tissue influences orthotic fit. The individual who has atrophy of the torso will need an orthosis that covers more area than does the person who has a normal amount of soft tissue.

Snug Fit

Regardless of material or design, some portion of an orthosis must touch the body. The contact should be snug, rather than constricting. An excessively tight band will compress superficial blood vessels and cause pain and abrasions. Equally important, the contact should not be loose. For example, an AFO that has an overly loose calf band will irritate the skin as the individual passes through the stance phase of gait.

Leverage

The longer the longitudinal segment of an orthosis, the less pressure exerted at each end to provide the same functional benefits. In a WHO, a relatively long forearm bar applies less pressure on the proximal forearm than a shorter bar. Excessive length, however, may impinge on the antecubital fossa, causing discomfort.

Orthotic Effectiveness

Although comfort is a prime prerequisite of all orthoses, the therapeutic benefit of the device will be realized only if the device applies forces effectively. An orthosis worn over a malaligned body segment can exert force to correct or reduce the deformity if the anatomic joint yields to passive force. If the deformity cannot be reduced passively, then the orthosis must accommodate the malalignment. For example, a patient may have a knee that rests in a position of genu valgum. When the clinician applies appropriate manual force, the knee achieves a straighter alignment. In such an instance, the patient would benefit from a corrective orthosis that will maintain the improved position. Alternatively, a person may have fixed bunion deformity that does not change when corrective force is exerted. The individual will benefit from an accommodative shoe that, although it does not change foot alignment, will be comfortable.

Pressure Systems

Supportive systems involve a series of forces and counterforces, which are known as pressure systems. The basic pressure system for an orthosis is the three-point force system. The system consists of a principal force acting in one direction and two counterforces acting in the opposite direction located proximal and distal to the principal force. For example, trunk flexion is controlled by an anteriorly directed force from the midportion of posterior uprights in a LS FEO (principal force) and posteriorly directed counterforces applied by the sternal plate and suprapubic plate (Figure 1-1a). Similarly, the patient who has genu valgum will have the deformity controlled by wearing a KAFO, which exerts laterally directed force on the medial aspect of the knee and medially directed counterforces on the lateral aspect of the thigh and leg (Figure 1-1b).

Some orthoses exert a four-point force system. The parapodium, a THKAFO, applies posteriorly directed forces from the chest band and the anterior leg bands, and also applies anteriorly directed forces from the dorsolumbar band and the back of the shoe supports (Figure 1-2).

In a few instances, the orthosis surrounds the body segment, applying circumferential total contact pressure. For example, the patient recovering from third-degree burns to the arm may be fitted with an elastic sleeve that distributes pressure over the greatest area.

Floor Reaction

The force exerted on the body in response to the force that the person exerts on the floor is called the floor or ground reaction force. It is equal in amount and opposite in direction to the force applied by the

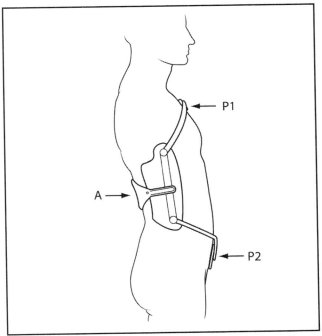

Figure 1-1a. Three-point pressure system in a lumbosacral flexion control orthosis to control trunk flexion. A = anteriorly directed force. P1 and P2 = posteriorly directed forces.

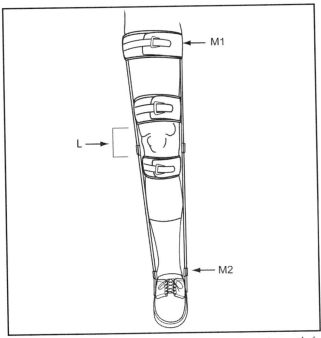

Figure 1-1b. Three-point pressure system in a left knee-ankle-foot orthosis to control genu valgum. L = laterally directed force. M1 and M2 = medially directed forces.

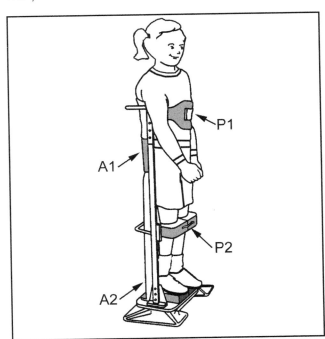

Figure 1-2. Four-point pressure system in a parapodium to assist standing. A1 and A2 = anteriorly directed forces. P1 and P2 = posteriorly directed forces.

patient. When one walks, the floor reaction is the resultant of the vertical force, which represents the interaction of gravity and acceleration; the horizontal force, which represents the tendency of the foot to slide forward; and the rotational force, which prevents the torsional movement of the leg. At the time of heel contact, the floor reaction normally passes behind the ankle, exerting a plantar flexion moment of force. Usually, contraction of the dorsiflexors controls ankle plantar flexion in response to this external force. All wearers of lower limb orthoses must contend with floor reactions while standing or during the stance phase of gait. The child who has cerebral palsy and who stands with crouched posture may benefit from a pair of AFOs, which resist ankle dorsiflexion by applying posteriorly directed force in the vicinity of the tibial tuberosity (Figure 1-3).

MATERIALS

Contemporary orthoses are constructed from a variety of materials. Orthoses often contain plastic and metal components and a few have leather, rubber, wood, or cloth elements. The physical and aesthetic properties of each material influence orthotic

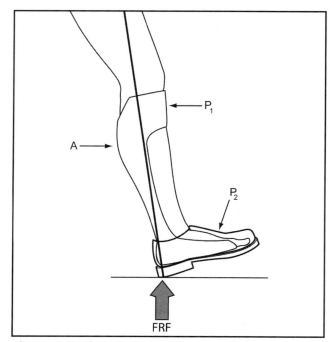

Figure 1-3. Three-point pressure system in an ankle-foot orthosis with solid ankle and anterior band. FRF = floor reaction force passing posterior to the ankle and through the knee axis. A = anteriorly directed force. P_1 = posteriorly directed force. P_2 = posteriorly directed force.

design, durability, and cost, as well as the patient's acceptance of the device. Materials differ in strength, flexibility, ease of forming, weight, and appearance.

Physical Characteristics

Certain physical characteristics pertain to all materials. The thicker a given material is, the more rigid, heavier, and bulkier the resulting orthosis. The shape of the material also influences its properties. An orthosis can be made stronger if its material is corrugated or curved, has rolled edges, or is reinforced. For example, carbon fiber can be embedded in plastic to enhance stiffness, or metal stays can be sewn into fabric to provide greater support. A given material that is shaped with an acute angle will bend more readily than the same material that has a more obtuse angle. This factor is especially important with regard to nicks and scratches in the orthosis. Breakage is more apt to occur at the site of the nick than in a smooth portion.

Strength

Strength is the ability of a material to resist forces. For example, an AFO for an adult with foot drop must be made of a stronger material than an AFO for a child with the same diagnosis because the forces exerted by a taller, heavier person are greater. Stress is the measure of force per unit area. Surface stress is called pressure. Great force over a small area causes high stress and high pressure. Orthoses must have sufficient strength to control stresses imposed by the wearer, and tissues must have good integrity to resist the pressure exerted by the orthosis.

Stress may be compressive, whereby force squeezes the material (Figure 1-4a); eg, an inflatable splint to stabilize a radial fracture sustained during a soccer game. Compressive stress enables pressure garments to control hypertrophic scarring in burned skin. Tensile stress, also known as distraction, involves pulling apart a material (Figure 1-4b). Examples include a coil spring in an AFO that provides dorsiflexion assistance by pulling the shoe upward during the swing phase of gait or a turnbuckle knee orthosis that passively stretches the joint capsule to reduce contracture. The third type of stress is shear, which is the horizontal sliding of one plane of the material over another (Figure 1-4c). Orthotic applications of shear are evident in the components of an overlapping joint in a WHO that exerts shear stress on one another or a knee orthosis that resists anterior gliding of the tibia over the femoral condyles or in trunk bracing to control a scoliotic curve.

Stress may result in strain, which is the change in the shape of a material. The amount of stress that must be applied to a material to cause strain is known as stiffness. Some orthoses utilize strain as part of their design. For example, the posterior leaf spring AFO is constructed from plastic that bends in response to ground reaction forces and resumes its original shape when force is removed. The solid construction of the orthosis with no mechanical joints allows the patient with weak dorsiflexors to achieve normal motion in both swing and stance phases of walking. Strain applied to a metal upright can shape it to fit the contours of a leg that has tibia varum. Similarly, strain on the medial aspect of a leather shoe's toe box can create a concavity to accommodate a painful bunion.

Material failure results from several causes. Excessive strain can deform an orthosis to the point where its clinical value is negated. For example, constant prolonged strain on a low-temperature plastic orthosis may change its shape so much that it no longer controls the body part for which it was made. A brittle material breaks when relatively low force is applied. Metal becomes more brittle when cold; therefore, more brace damage occurs in the winter. Leather becomes brittle when not regularly treated with saddle soap. Fatigue resistance is the ability of

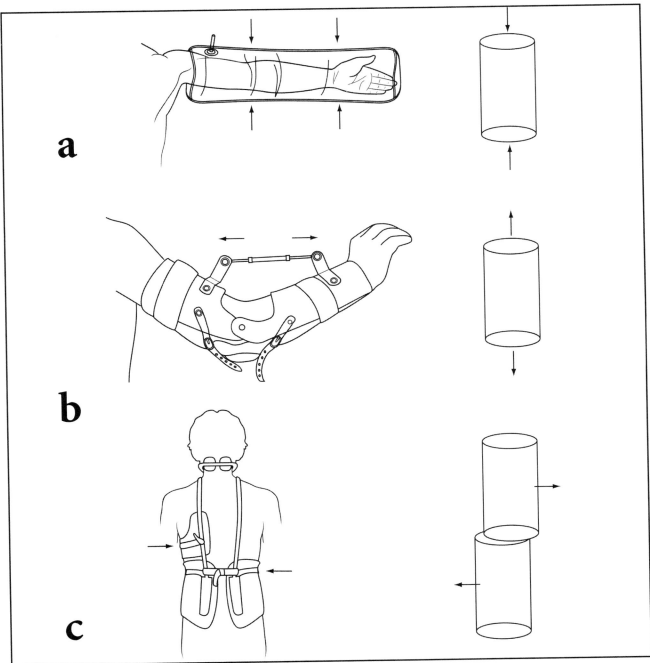

Figure 1-4a through c. Stresses: a. Compressive. b. Tensile. c. Shear.

the material to withstand cyclic loading. An active child, for example, subjects his orthosis to much repetitive loading; consequently, the metal joints may eventually fail and necessitate frequent repairs.

Other Properties

Other properties of materials used in orthoses include elasticity, plasticity, malleability, and corrosion resistance. Elasticity is the ratio of stress to strain; ie, the ability of a material to recover its original dimensions (eg, rubber-reinforced canvas in a corset accommodates to changes in contour of the torso as the patient moves from standing to sitting). Plasticity characterizes a material that changes shape without cracking. Plasticity is evident in a malleable material such as a polyethylene foam resilient insole, which reshapes under compression. Ductile materials also exhibit plasticity (eg, wire alters shape under tension). Corrosion resistance refers to the extent to which materials deteriorate when exposed to chemicals. For some patients, orthoses are vulnerable to urine and perspiration, which attack the structure of the material, particularly certain metals and some fabrics.

Material properties influence orthotic prescription in many ways. An AFO made of relatively thin polyethylene would suffice for a child with cerebral palsy. If the patient were an adult with comparable spasticity, thicker plastic would be more appropriate. Another child with severe equinovarus might have an orthosis of similar design reinforced with medial and lateral carbon fiber inserts.

Plastic

All plastics are synthetic organic (carbon-containing) materials. The enormous variety of plastics indicates the many ways in which the molecules of the constituent elements can be combined. Simple chemical units, such as ethylene, are called monomers. Most orthoses, however, are made of complex chemical units, which are called polymers, such as polyethylene. Molecular arrangement dictates the properties of the plastic. As a group, plastics are relatively lightweight, easily shaped, strong, easily cleaned, corrosion resistant, and available in many colors.[3,4]

Thermoplastics

Many orthoses are made of thermoplastic. When heated, the material becomes malleable and can be reshaped. Upon cooling, the material retains the new shape. Usually, the plastic can be reheated and reshaped indefinitely, thus permitting the orthotist to alter the fit of the appliance by heating the plastic, as well as by removing or adding material.[5] Some thermoplastics become malleable at relatively low heat. WHOs are usually formed from plastics that become malleable when immersed in warm water. These plastics are convenient to make orthoses quickly because the warm plastic can be molded directly on the patient's hand or other body segment. Unfortunately, if the person who wears a WHO made of such plastic washes dishes in warm water, the orthosis may change shape. Some thermoplastics require heating to a high temperature to become malleable. These plastics are usually formed over a plaster model of the body part.[6,7] Many thermoplastics are relatively weak, retain soil, and are flammable.[8]

When resilience is desired in an orthosis, the clinician can select an open- or closed-cell thermoplastic. The manufacturer creates sponginess in the material by forcing nitrogen or other gas into the plastic. Resilient materials are available in various degrees of compressibility, as well as in several thicknesses and colors.

Thermosets

Alternate molecular arrangements produce thermosetting plastics such as polyester. Once molded, the plastic cannot be reshaped. An orthosis made of thermosetting plastic is virtually impervious to heat but can only be altered by grinding or cutting material from the plastic or by adding pads.

Plastics and similar materials used in orthoses, as well as their characteristics, are listed in Table 1-1.

Metal

A metal is a chemical element that is lustrous, opaque, fusible, and ductile. Some elements, particularly carbon and silicone, are intermediate between metals and nonmetals and are known as metalloids. Most metals are used in alloys, which are a combination of elements, at least one of which is a metal. Alloys improve strength, wear resistance, and corrosion resistance. The mechanical properties of metals depend on their chemical structure. As a group, metals are strong, stiff, fatigue-resistant, and impervious to the effects of environmental heat.[9]

Steel

Steel in orthoses is usually stainless steel, which is an alloy of iron, nickel, and chromium. Nickel increases corrosion resistance; chromium makes the metal more ductile. Stainless steel is heavier, stiffer, and stronger than most other materials. Because it is radiopaque, steel is undesirable if the patient with scoliosis requires periodic radiographs while wearing the orthosis.

Aluminum

Aluminum is often alloyed with copper, manganese, and other elements. When compared with steel, aluminum is more malleable and one-third as heavy. Thus, to achieve equivalent rigidity, the aluminum components of an orthosis have to be bulkier. Aluminum, which is radiolucent, is more subject to fatigue failure than steel. These qualities make aluminum unsuitable for orthotic joints.

Titanium

Titanium is very lightweight and corrosion resistant, making it desirable for orthotic joints. It is more expensive than steel or aluminum, so it is used less often.

TABLE 1-1

Plastics Used in Orthotic Fabrication

Generic Name	Brand Name	Characteristics	Comments
Polyethylene	Ortholen	Easy to form, flexible, lightweight, good resistance to fatigue and chemicals	Used where great strength is not required (eg, most AFOs)
Polyethylene foam	Plastazote, Pelite, Aliplast, and Dermaplast	Closed cellular structure that is resilient, very lightweight, and flexible	Suitable for padding and lining straps and in shock-absorbing FOs; eventually, the cells compress ("bottom out")
Polyethylene foam alloy, ethylene vinyl acetate	Nickelplast	Denser than polyethylene foam	Resists bottoming out
Polypropylene	None	Durable, but more difficult to form	A stiffer thermoplastic, used where greater strength is needed, such as KAFOs
Copolymer	None	More fracture-resistant and durable than polypropylene, but more difficult to form	A blend of polypropylene and polyethylene
Polyolefin	Surlyn	Easier to form than pure polyethylene	Has good optical clarity so the orthosis is less conspicuous
Ethylene vinyl acetate (EVA)	None	Polyolefin copolymer, which is lightweight with excellent shock absorbency	Often used in shoes
Acrylic	Plexidur and Nyloplex	Rigid plastics	Usually polymerized from methyl-methacrylate polymers; acrylic is available in transparent form
Transpolyisoprene	Orthoplast and Ezeform	Rubbery thermoplastic formable at low temperature	Used principally for upper-limb orthoses where low force will be applied by the patient
Polycaprolactone	Polyform and Orthoplast II	A more rigid thermoplastic, which can be formed on the patient	Suitable for upper-limb and trunk orthoses
Polyurethane elastomer	Sorbothane, Viscolas, and PQ	Relatively heavy and difficult to cut	Exhibits good dampening property, comparable to the viscoelasticity of muscle
Polyurethane foam	Poron, Sorbothane, and Ovafit	Does not stretch appreciably	Has open-cell composition, suiting it for some foot orthoses

Table 1-1 (Continued)			
Generic Name	Brand Name	Characteristics	Comments
Nylon	Zytel	Semirigid plastic	Well-suited for orthotic joints, which are lighter in weight than metal ones
Polyester resin	None	Used to permeate fabric to create a rigid or semirigid laminate	Useful for the shells of lower-limb orthoses
Carbon fiber	Graphite	Ultra lightweight and very durable but expensive and difficult to cut	Used to reinforce portions of the orthosis that will be subjected to great stress; for example, the medial and lateral sides of an AFO may have carbon fiber insets to resist any tendency of the wearer to pronate or supinate the foot
Silicone	Silipos	Excellent friction resistance	May be combined with fabric for liners and pads

Leather

Leather is animal skin that is chemically treated in the process known as tanning. The skin is soaked in a solution usually composed of natural or synthetic vegetable products or chromium. The process toughens the skin and makes it more flexible, stronger, and more porous. The specific skin and the type of tanning determine the flexibility, durability, and appearance of the leather. Leather is porous, does not compress, and can be molded over a model of the body part. If the patient is allergic to a particular leather, the contact dermatitis may be resolved with another leather, a fabric interface between the leather and the patient's skin, or a hypoallergenic plastic or fabric substitute.

Cowhide is exceptionally strong and is widely used for straps and the upper portion of shoes. Horsehide frequently lines bands, such as a calf band or thigh band, because its texture is particularly comfortable next to the skin. Kidskin and deerskin in shoe uppers suit patients who have hammer toes and other tender areas.

Wood

The most common wood used in orthoses is cork. The bark of the cork oak tree is exceptionally lightweight and resilient, and is used primarily for shoe lifts and arch supports. Sometimes, cork is ground and mixed with rubber or other materials to achieve greater flexibility or economy. Cushion cork is a combination of cork and rubber. Thermocork (Apex Foot Health Industries, Inc, Teaneck, NJ) or Birko Cork (Birkenstock, Novato, Calif) is a composite of cork and thermoplastic material. Other woods are occasionally used in shoe construction. For example, balsa is appreciably lighter than cork, yet it has comparable strength and resilience, so shoe elevations are sometimes made of balsa wood.

Rubber

The sap of rubber trees is cured to form rubber, which is noted for its elasticity, shock absorbency, and toughness. Synthetic rubber, such as neoprene, is less expensive and more resistant to corrosion. Whether natural or synthetic, rubber provides excellent traction on shoe soles and is a good padding material. Rubber strands may be woven with cotton or other fabric to create elastic straps. Spenco (Apex Foot Health Industries, Inc, Teaneck, NJ) is a closed-cell expanded rubber manufactured by introducing nitrogen gas into neoprene. As the gas expands it forms many closed cells. The material has excellent shock absorbency and shear force resistance. Lynco (Apex Foot Health Industries, Inc, Teaneck, NJ) and Kemblo (Pel Supply Company, Cleveland, Ohio) are examples of sponge rubber. Sodium bicarbonate is forced into rubber, creating an open-cell structure. Such rubber is softer and more porous than other types of rubber. Latex foam is another example of open-cell rubber. It is washable, soft, and very resilient, although the cells compress permanently after a relatively brief period of repetitive use.

Fabric

Cotton, wool, and synthetic materials are commonly found in orthoses. The properties of the fabric depend on the material itself and the way in which the material is formed.

Cotton

Cotton is strong, absorbs perspiration readily, and is hypoallergenic. Consequently, cotton canvas is desirable for the sturdy abdominal front on a trunk orthosis. Canvas forms a porous shoe upper, which is part of many athletic shoes. Cotton flannel is a good padding material, particularly for the metal components of a trunk orthosis. Knitted cotton conforms readily to the body and is often used as a liner under a leg or trunk orthosis.[10]

Wool

Wool is relatively expensive but has excellent resiliency. Wool felt is used in certain foot orthoses and cervical orthoses. Felt is a fabric made from wool and other fibers matted together by steam and pressure. The higher the wool content, the more durable the felt. Felt is lightweight and porous but compresses readily.

Synthetic Fabrics

Synthetic fabrics used in orthoses include polyester and nylon. Polyester fibers may be combined with cotton to create a relatively inexpensive material that is strong and dries easily. A corset made of polyester and cotton will not retain perspiration as much as one made entirely of cotton. A very popular use of nylon is hook-and-pile fasteners, which are easier to engage than buckles, snaps, buttons, or laces.

Fabric may incorporate rubber to create an elastic cloth useful for straps and for portions of the orthosis, such as a trunk orthosis, which should yield when the wearer moves. Elastic fabrics are used in pressure garments to control edema, provide some joint stability, and prevent hypertrophic scarring.

Adhesive

In some orthoses, such as foot orthoses, two materials must be attached to one another. Rather than use mechanical means, such as rivets or thread, the materials may be glued. Because adhesion depends on the chemical characteristics of the surfaces to be joined, no universal adhesive exists. Synthetic resins, whether thermoplastic or thermosetting, are widely used in orthotics because of their ability to bond many surfaces, such as joining a strap to the shell of a wrist-hand orthosis. Rubber-based adhesives have great resistance to impact loads, making them very suitable for many applications in foot orthoses. Protein adhesives (either animal or vegetable), while excellent for joining wood and paper, are less commonly used in orthotics. Some adhesives are toxic or flammable and are unsuitable for pediatric orthoses.

CONSTRUCTION METHODS

Orthoses are made in various ways. Many are mass-produced. The clinician can select from a vast array of products, such as corsets or hand splints, and choose the one appliance that will best suit a given patient. Often, the clinician adjusts the mass-produced orthosis so that it fits the patient precisely. Such customizing can result in a relatively inexpensive, readily available orthosis, shortening the delay between prescription and delivery of a finished device.

Custom-made orthoses can be made by molding sheet plastic directly on the body, as is often done with hand orthoses. The plastic is then trimmed and straps and other accessories are attached.

Other custom-made orthoses involve more elaborate methods. The orthotist wraps the body part in plaster to form a negative model of the part. After the plaster sets, it is removed from the body. The next step is to pour liquid plaster into the hollow model to create a positive, solid model. Usually the model is modified. Portions that will be in contact with sensitive areas have reliefs, created by adding material to the positive model, which, in turn, will create a slight concavity in the plastic, which is molded over the model. Conversely, areas in contact with fleshy parts, which tolerate loading very well, will have material removed from the positive model. The resulting orthosis has a slight convexity ("build-up") at that point (eg, a trunk orthosis will have reliefs over the iliac crests and a build-up over the abdomen).

Orthoses with metal uprights are usually made from a pattern, which the orthotist designs by taking linear and circumferential measurements of the limb. Factory-made uprights are individually bent and are attached to custom-made plastic, leather, or upholstered metal bands and shells.

Computer-aided design and computer-aided manufacture (CAD-CAM) is the newest mode of fabrication. The body part is exposed to an electronic sensor, such as a laser scanner, which creates a detailed pattern of the segment. A computer program then refines the initial pattern to exaggerate loading on pressure-tolerant areas and minimize load on sensitive structures. Fabrication usually involves electronic creation of a positive model over which plastic is formed. CAD-CAM enables fabrication of the orthosis at a site distant from the place in which the patient's part was scanned. The system also facilitates storage and retrieval of detailed information about the patient's contours.

SUMMARY

Orthoses are orthopedic appliances used to support, align, prevent, or correct deformities of a body part or to improve the function of movable parts of the body. Key members of the orthotic clinic team include the patient, orthotist, physician, and physical therapist. Others, such as a pedorthist, occupational therapist, social worker, and psychologist, may contribute valuable insights into the team's deliberations. The team formulates the orthotic prescription and is responsible for the patient's use of the orthosis. In addition to the patient's biomechanical requirements, the team considers the individual's goals, psychosocial status, previous orthotic experience, and preferences. Other factors influencing the prescription are the duration of anticipated wear, the environment in which the orthosis will be worn, financial resources, and the patient's hand function and visual acuity.

Current nomenclature emphasizes a generic approach. For example, ankle-foot orthosis (AFO) is preferred to such terms as club foot brace or Scarpa's boot. Trunk orthoses are designed by the region encompassed by the orthosis and the motions controlled; thus, a lumbosacral flexion-extension control orthosis (LS FEO) restricts flexion and extension of the low back. Similarly, upper-limb orthoses have generic names. Orthoses have been worn for many centuries. The names of some pioneers, such as Thomas and Hessing, are occasionally used today to designate particular appliances.

The biomechanical purposes of orthoses are fundamentally resisting or assisting motion, transferring load from one bodily structure to another, or protecting a body part. Regardless of purpose, the orthosis must be comfortable. Three-point and other pressure systems enable the orthosis to provide the desired support. The distance between the contact points influences the patient's comfort.

Plastics, metals, leathers, and other materials are used in contemporary orthoses. All materials exhibit some degree of strength, flexibility, weight, elasticity, plasticity, and corrosion resistance. The clinic team selects the material according to the properties most appropriate for the given patient. Orthoses may be mass-produced or custom-made in a variety of procedures.

THOUGHT QUESTIONS

1. The patient has diabetic neuropathy, which has resulted in foot dragging during the swing phase of gait. What health care providers are most directly concerned with prescribing an orthosis for this individual?

2. How would the prescription of an AFO for the patient in Question 1 differ if the patient were homeless as compared with the prescription if the individual were a computer programmer?

3. Discuss the factors that contribute to creating a comfortable orthosis.

4. Name two circumstances when an aluminum and leather KAFO would be preferable to a polypropylene and carbon fiber orthosis.

REFERENCES

1. *Dorland's Illustrated Medical Dictionary.* 28th ed. Philadelphia, Pa: WB Saunders Company; 1994:1194.

2. Gibson T, Wilson E. The history of orthotics. In: Murdoch G, ed. *The Advance in Orthotics.* London: Edward Arnold; 1976:1-14.

3. Clover W. Lower extremity thermoplastics: an overview. *Journal of Prosthetics and Orthotics.* 1991;3:9-13.

4. Lunsford T. The properties of plastics. *Biomechanics.* 1995;12:50-61.

5. Oberg K. Cost-benefits in orthopaedic technology by using thermoplastics in developing countries. *Prosthet Orthot Int.* 1991;15:18-22.

6. Pritham CH. Thermoplastics in lower extremity prosthetics: equipment, components, and techniques. *Journal of Prosthetics and Orthotics.* 1991;3:14-21.

7. Schuch CM. Thermoplastic applications in lower extremity plastics. *Journal of Prosthetics and Orthotics.* 1991;3:1-8.

8. Compton J, Edelstein JE. New plastics for forming directly on the patient. *Prosthet Orthot Int.* 1978;2:43-47.

9. American Academy of Orthopaedic Surgeons. *Orthopaedic Appliances Atlas.* Vol 1. Ann Arbor, Mich: JW Edwards; 1952:1-16.

10. Sanders JE, Green JM, Mitchell SB, Zachariah SG. Material properties of commonly-used interface materials and their static coefficients of friction with skin and sockets. *J Rehabil Res Dev.* 1998;35:161-176.

RECOMMENDED READING

1. Armesto DG, Lehneis HR, Frisina W. Orthotics design with advanced materials and methods: a pilot study. *Rehabilitation Research and Development Progress Reports.* Baltimore, Md: Department of Veterans Affairs; 1997:215-216.

2. Kuncir EJ, Wirta RW, Golbranson FL. Load-bearing characteristics of polyethylene foam: an examination of structural and compression properties. *J Rehabil Res Dev.* 1990;27:229-238.

3. Stallard J. Lower limb orthotics. In: Dvir Z, ed. *Clinical Biomechanics.* New York, NY: Churchill Livingstone; 2000:239-266.

Chapter 2

Foot Orthoses

"How lovely are thy feet with shoes, oh prince's daughter."
Song of Songs 4:1

Virtually all people wear shoes. When prescribed for therapeutic purposes, shoes may be considered foot orthoses. As is true with every orthosis, the shoe applies force. Shoes are often modified by the addition of material applied on the outer sole or inside the shoe, which alters the forces that the shoe applies. The responsibility of the orthotic clinical team is to select the most appropriate footwear for a particular patient so that the individual may enjoy improved function when standing and walking.

This chapter considers shoes from a clinical perspective. Shoes that are appropriate for patients with foot discomfort, deformity, and disease are analyzed. Orthotic interventions for the most common disorders are presented, as are suggestions for examining and obtaining models of the feet. Evaluation of foot orthoses and their maintenance are included in Chapter 6, Evaluation Procedures for Lower-Limb Orthoses.

HISTORICAL PERSPECTIVE

From prehistoric bulrush, grass, and leather moccasins[1] to Cinderella's glass slippers and Dorothy's ruby pumps in *The Wizard of Oz*, shoes have been part of history and legend.[2,3] In some cultures, modesty dictates that women's feet remain unseen, covered with the finest shoes that the household can afford. Shoes have always indicated social rank. Historically, limited mobility was viewed as aristocratic. A particularly egregious example is Chinese foot-binding, which was practiced from the 10th century to 1911 on girls as young as 4 years old. The resulting lily-pad feet compelled a mincing, painful gait.[4] Women with small feet remain culturally desirable to the present day. Some aspects of modern fashion reflect historic peculiarities. For example, in 16th century Venice, platforms as high as 27 inches were in vogue. Contemporary platform soles and heels, stiletto heels, triangular toe boxes, and improper shoe size compel wearers to seek medical attention to address pain, sprain, fracture, and other disorders.

Modern shoe production originated in the 19th century. Invention of sewing and riveting machines changed the way most Americans and Europeans obtained shoes. Mass production eclipsed the custom shoemaker, obliging most people to choose from styles and shapes determined by unseen factory owners. The same century also saw the introduction of left and right shoes and the present system of full and half sizes.

Shoe Styles

Although shoes are manufactured in a vast array of designs and materials, they are all designed to protect the plantar surface of the foot from abrasions and lacerations that might otherwise be caused by the walking surface. In addition, shoes usually shield the toes from stubbing and provide protection from inclement weather. Shoes are often considered a fashion accessory; consequently, shoes that are not stylish or are termed "orthopedic" have a negative connotation.[5] Although "orthopedic shoe" connotes a sturdy, laced shoe that may suit many patients with foot deformity or paralysis, the term usually designates shoes that are relatively expensive and unattractive. Consequently, rather than being designated as "orthopedic," the shoes described in this chapter will be described by their pertinent features. The clinician should indicate the particular characteristics of the shoe that are pertinent to the given patient's requirements.

Most feet can be accommodated with mass-produced shoes. They are less expensive than custom-made ones and are available without a waiting period. In contrast, custom-made shoes require several weeks for their construction. Unless the foot is markedly deformed, custom-made shoes are unnecessary.

PARTS OF SHOES

The major parts of a shoe are the upper, sole, heel, and reinforcements (Figure 2-1). Each component of a shoe can contribute to its therapeutic value.

Upper

The portion of the shoe that covers the dorsal aspect of the foot and encases the heel is the upper. A major consideration when selecting shoes is the upper's appearance. For the patient with foot deformity or pain, the upper can either accommodate or irritate tender areas. For example, a foot with claw toes, hammer toes, or dorsal corns requires a shoe with an upper that has a spacious toe box, such as a moccasin style. The extra-depth shoe has an upper that is more spacious than that of an ordinary shoe and can accommodate an insert, a deformed foot, or a plaster or bandage dressing.

The person who has chronic edema should not wear shoes that have narrow straps, which would concentrate pressure. An open-back, "sling-back" shoe imposes high pressure on the back of the heel.

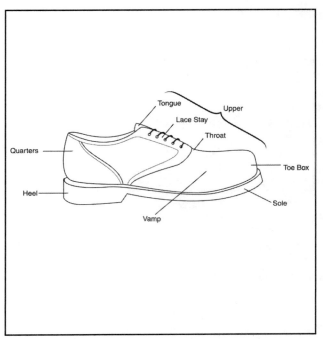

Figure 2-1. Parts of a shoe.

Height

The height of the upper may be a clinical consideration. Most patients are well served by a low upper. An oxford shoe has a low upper with laced closure (Figure 2-2). The low upper terminates distal to the malleoli. A shoe with a high upper (Figure 2-3) is sometimes referred to as a boot or bootie and is indicated when mediolateral support is required. The high upper can contribute to the stability of the hind- and midfoot; however, if the patient is wearing an ankle-foot orthosis (AFO), which provides such support, a high upper is not necessary. A high shoe may be needed to encase a foot with marked Achilles' contracture or a foot with forefoot or midfoot amputation. As compared with high shoes, low ones are less restrictive, easier to don, and less expensive. A collar added to the top of the upper converts a low shoe into a high one; this alteration is particularly useful for the patient who has hemiparesis with pes equinus.

Closure

The mode of closing the upper may be a clinically important issue. Laces, preferably drawn through four or five pairs of eyelets, provide the greatest range of girth adjustability. The patient who is not dexterous will be better served with straps secured by buckles or hook-and-pile tape. The individual with hemiparesis should have the strap on the paretic side pull toward the nonparetic side. Another

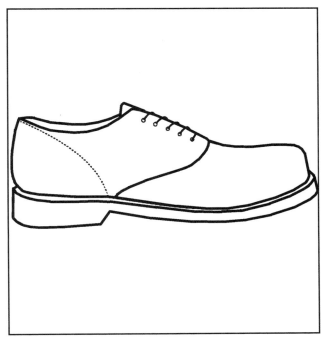

Figure 2-2. Low upper.

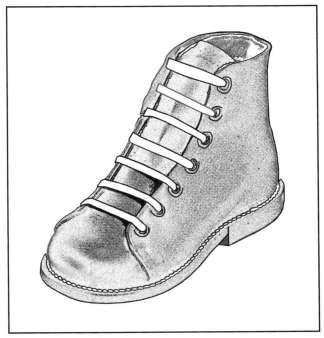

Figure 2-3. High upper.

alternative to laces is a flap with a hook and pile surface, although it is more difficult to achieve snug fit with this closure. The shoe worn with an insert AFO, such as a posterior leaf spring orthosis, should have a lace or strap closure high on the dorsum of the foot.

Throat Styles

The shoe's closure is attached to the upper at the throat. Throat styles are distinguished by the design of the anterior margin of the closure. The most versatile type of throat style is the Blucher (Figure 2-4), which has a loose anterior margin of the lace stays. It was named for Blucher, a Prussian general in the Franco-Prussian War. This design, also known as "open lacing,"[6] enables the wearer to fold the shoe's tongue back to create the largest opening into the shoe. This may be important in the presence of toe deformities or for donning an orthosis that has a shoe insert. The Blucher throat also has maximum adjustability. An alternative is the Bal or Balmoral throat style (Figure 2-5), which has the anterior margins of the lace stays sewn together. Its name refers to Balmoral Castle, which is owned by the British royal family. The Bal style, also called "closed lacing," provides a narrower opening into the shoe.

Material

The material of the upper is another potential prescription issue. Leather is the traditional material because it can be easily molded and readily cleaned.

Suppler than calfskin, kidskin and deerskin suit the patient with dorsal corns. Canvas has a porous structure, which provides ventilation for the foot. Nylon is lightweight, is porous, and minimizes friction. Elastic materials, such as neoprene and spandex or Lycra, provide a snugger, more secure fit. The patient with severe toe deformities will be best served with a shoe that has a high toe box or one that has the leather upper treated chemically so that it can be heat-shaped.

Sole

The sole is the portion of the shoe that lies under the plantar surface of the foot. The shoe which has both an inner and outer sole is easier to modify. The extra-depth shoe has two inner soles. The upper one can be removed to provide room for an insert, foot dressings, or foot deformities. Athletic shoes sometimes have a midsole interposed between the insole and the outsole. The midsole may be made of foam polymer to increase shock absorption and stability. A leather outer sole is easy to modify; however, a rubber sole can be altered with modern adhesives without difficulty. The rubber sole provides greater traction than the leather version and, depending on the type of rubber, may contribute to shock absorption[7] and pain relief.[8] Rubber soles may have ripples, waffle designs, or studs to increase traction.

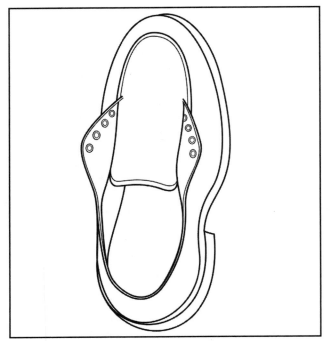

Figure 2-4. Blucher throat style.

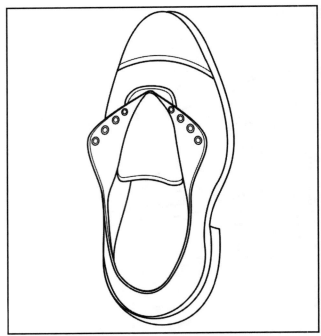

Figure 2-5. Bal throat style.

Heel

The shoe heel lies under the anatomic heel. Heel height is usually measured in 1/8-inch increments. A man's dress heel is 6/8 or 7/8 inch. The higher the heel, the more weight is shifted to the forefoot.[9,10] Because the high heel interferes with balance and its small base offers little traction, the individual is at greater risk for falling when wearing a shoe with a spike heel as compared with wearing a tennis shoe. The high curved heel of a cowboy boot is associated with greater likelihood of falling as compared with low heeled shoes.[11] Healthy adults wearing 2 1/2-inch heels use more muscular effort to maintain balance than when wearing flat-heeled shoes.[12] Long-term wearing of high-heeled shoes permits the Achilles' tendon to shorten. Shoes with heels higher than 3 inches displace substantial load to the forefoot, aggravating metatarsalgia, hammer toes, and bunions.[13] The forefoot deformities are exaggerated by a shoe that has a triangular toe box or an open toe.

Some clinicians claim that wearing high-heeled shoes contributes to an increased lumbar lordosis, but research has not supported this view.[14]

Occasionally, a higher heel is indicated. For example, the patient with heel pain will be more comfortable with anterior weight transfer. The patient with pes equinus or a short leg will usually walk with less deviation if the shoe has a heel lift or a higher heel.

One innovative heel includes a coiled spring system, which reduces impact during early stance (Figure 2-6).

Reinforcements

Heel Counter

The three major reinforcements are the heel counter, the shank, and the toe box (Figure 2-7). The heel counter stiffens the posterior portion of the upper that covers the anatomic heel. The counter withstands high torsional forces, increases stability, and reduces the speed of hindfoot pronation. For the patient with heel spur, for example, the counter should fit snugly to prevent heel abrasion. Ordinarily, the medial and lateral ends of the counter lie at the anterior border of the heel. Sometimes the counter extends farther forward. For example, a child with marked pes planus may be fitted with a shoe having a long medial counter. An adult with hyperpronation and instability may also benefit from a shoe with a long medial counter.

Shank

The shank (see Figure 2-7) is the longitudinal reinforcement of the midportion of the shoe. The shoe that is to be worn with a stirrup attachment for an AFO should have a steel shank so that the rivets securing the stirrup may be firmly embedded.

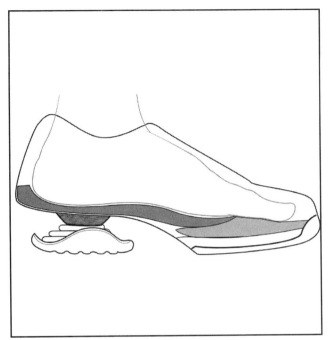

Figure 2-6. Heel with a coiled spring.

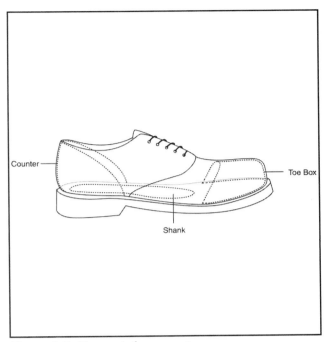

Figure 2-7. Shoe reinforcements.

Toe Box

The toe box (see Figure 2-7) shields the toes from trauma such as stubbing or injury if an object was dropped on the forefoot. The toe box should not contact the dorsum of the foot. The patient with toe deformity should have a shoe with a high toe box. Similarly, some athletes require a spacious toe box. A long-distance runner may need an extra inch to accommodate the swelling that occurs during marathons.

Last

The last (Figure 2-8) is the model over which the shoe is made, even though it is not visible in the finished shoe. The last determines the three-dimensional shape of the shoe, including the contour of the toe box and counter, the space inside the shoe, and the heel height. Shoe fit depends on the size and configuration of the last, rather than just the shoe size, which only designates length and width. Typical lasts are described as regular (shaped like the foot), straight (with little curvature), curved, inflared, and outflared (Figure 2-9). An inflared last provides more room medially, while a shoe made over an outflared last accommodates forefoot abductus. The patient with severe bunions will achieve greater comfort in a shoe made over a bunion last, which provides additional medial roominess.

SPECIAL-PURPOSE SHOES

Shoes for patients with foot pain are frequently referred to as comfort or walking shoes. Typically, these shoes have especially spacious toe boxes to accommodate swelling, which normally occurs in the late afternoon after a full day's wearing. Comfort shoes often have laced or strap closures to help stabilize the foot. They also have resilient material in the insole or outsole, or in both areas. Some comfort shoes have a second removable insole placed over the primary insole. The removable insole can be replaced by a custom-made insert.

For individuals whose feet differ in size, there are three ways to achieve good fit for each foot: a) one pair of split-size shoes, b) two pairs of shoes, with the unneeded shoes discarded, and c) one pair of shoes—the larger foot will be well-fitted in one shoe, while the smaller foot will be placed in a shoe that has a custom-made insert to occupy the superfluous space. Split-size shoes are relatively expensive and are available in a limited number of styles and colors. Two pairs of shoes allow the wearer the widest range of style and color but at double the price each time shoes are purchased. The third option, while expensive initially, enables the wearer to purchase ordinary shoes, assuming all shoes have been made over the same last. The insert can be transferred from one shoe to the next.

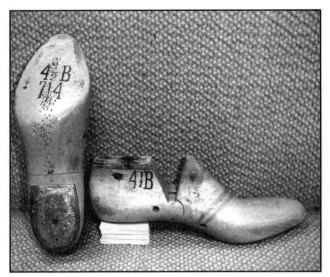

Figure 2-8. Last.

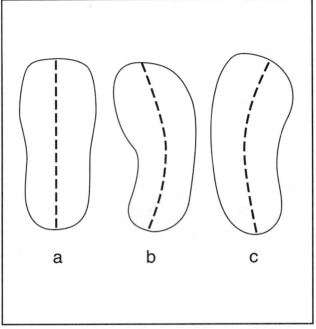

Figure 2-9. Children's last types for a right shoe. a. Straight. b. Inflared. c. Outflared.

Infants and young children do not need shoes for standing or walking. Socks may be worn for warmth. Toddlers' shoes should have smooth soles to make walking easy. Heavy or high-friction soles can cause falls. A bootie is useful because it reduces the likelihood that the infant or toddler will take the shoe off the foot. Foot orthoses are rarely indicated inasmuch as those younger than 16 months have flat feet, and the longitudinal arch is not fully developed until approximately 7 years of age. Juvenile feet grow in spurts. Youngsters from 16 to 24 months of age usually grow half a shoe size every 3 months, while children over 3 years of age increase an average of half a size every 4 to 6 months. Most children require relatively wide shoes. Lacing enables the easiest adjustment for a snug fit.

Shoes intended for long-distance walking and hiking should be spacious in the toe area and should have a shock-absorbent, preferably wedged, sole to ease transition through stance phase. The upper should be porous for ventilation. A high upper contributes to ankle support, which is desirable for walking on uneven terrain. A firm counter and a rigid shank provide support to accommodate the demands of long-distance walking.

Athletic shoes are appropriate for many children and adults who have foot disorders.[15] Such shoes have a shock-absorbing rubber sole. They can be opened widely to ease donning, especially if the individual has an insert orthosis. Both canvas and leather

uppers are porous, making the footwear cooler. In addition, patients usually are pleased with the fashionable appearance of athletic shoes and are thus more compliant with the therapeutic program.

Different sports are played with different shoes, which have specific features. Most athletic shoes have a resilient midsole interposed between the insole and the outsole. A polyurethane midsole is more durable but heavier than an ethylene vinyl acetate one. Running shoes should have a resilient sole that tilts up from the ground and is flexible enough to permit at least 25 degrees of metatarsophalangeal hyperextension.[16] The toe box should be round and high enough to prevent toe injury. A studded or waffle sole provides more traction and shock absorption than a smooth sole. The heel counter should be firm and well-padded to stabilize the heel. The heel should have a 1/2 inch elevation to reduce stress on the Achilles' tendon. Aerobic exercise shoes should be lightweight with extra resilience under the forefoot. Tennis (or court) shoes should provide mediolateral stability and have a flexible sole to facilitate quick forward movements. The shoe sole material should provide sufficient traction. Court surfaces vary; therefore, the sole material should be selected appropriately. Field shoes, intend-

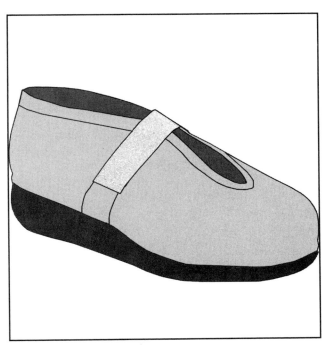

Figure 2-10. Healing shoe.

ed for baseball, football, soccer, and similar sports, have fixed or detachable cleats to maximize traction on earthen and grassy fields. Basketball shoes have a thick, stiff sole for extra stability when running and a high top to promote ankle stability. Cross-training shoes have a flexible forefoot with mediolateral hindfoot control. Shoes for skiing, skating, and dance should fit very snugly so they provide minimal room for an insert.[17-19]

Patients with diabetic ulcers may be provided with healing shoes (Figure 2-10), which have a resilient wedge sole and a polyethylene foam upper for temporary wear.[20] The upper can be heat-modified with the shoe off the foot, thereby accommodating foot deformities or bulky dressings. Custom-molded inserts are especially beneficial for patients with sensory deficit.[21,22] The federal Therapeutic Shoe Bill passed in May 1993 provides Medicare reimbursement for therapeutic shoes to people with diabetes.

Sandals are an alternative to closed shoes and may be useful for patients who have marked toe deformities. Sandals offer necessary ventilation in very hot climates. An AFO can be worn with a sturdy sandal that has a strap high on the dorsum of the foot. The strap design determines the areas of pressure concentration. Broad straps are essential to avoiding undue pressure. Sandals, however, offer virtually no protection against stubbing the toes or other trauma to the dorsum of the foot.

FOOT EXAMINATION

Inspection of the foot (Table 2-1) should include examination of the skin to detect abrasions, lacerations, and other blemishes.[23] Toe deformities should be noted because either the deformities will have to be reduced or the shoe will have to accommodate them. The skin between toes deserves special attention because infections are more likely to develop in the confined moist area of the dorsum than in the open area of the dorsum. Abnormally cool feet indicate vascular deficiency, while excessive warmth is associated with infection. The nails should be trimmed straight across to avoid infection. Plantar callosity indicates areas of high pressure and friction, which are vulnerable to pain due to overloading and infection if bacteria accumulate in the fissures of the callus. Sensory deficits can be detected with the use of monofilaments.[24] The examiner shields the patient's eyes, presses the filament on specific sites (Figure 2-11), and asks the patient where touch has occurred.

An imprint of the patient's weight-bearing pattern provides the clinician with information about plantar forces. The imprint may be made quickly and inexpensively with a Harris mat (Figure 2-12). The mat is a rubber grid slightly larger than a large foot. The clinician inks the grid, places a sheet of paper over the grid, and puts the mat on the floor. For a static imprint, the patient stands barefoot on the mat, while the clinician traces the outline of the floor. For a dynamic imprint, the patient walks barefoot onto it. In either instance, the resulting imprint indicates areas of relatively high and low pressure concentration and yields insight into areas at risk for ulceration. The tracing is useful to compare with the outline of the patient's shoe. Not uncommonly, the older patient will be wearing a shoe that is too small. As one ages, the foot elongates and widens in response to ligamentous laxity. Foot proportions also change. The heel, composed only of the calcaneus, remains essentially the same size, while the forefoot, with its many bones and ligaments, demonstrates the most alteration in width, length, and height.

Other means of documenting foot loading are insoles or mats equipped with pressure sensors that are connected to a computer. As the subject walks, the monitor displays load patterns in colors corresponding to various pressures or images that show peaks and valleys of loading. Electronic mats and insoles can reveal areas of incipient overloading and are especially useful for patients who have diabetes.[25]

Table 2-1

Checklist for Foot Inspection

- Skin: color, texture, moisture, temperature, mobility, lesions, sensation
- Hair: quality, distribution
- Nails: color, thickness, deformities (pits, grooves), redness
- Osseous or soft tissue deformities, such as bunions, subluxed fat pads, Charcot's joints
- Talocrural, subtalar, metatarsophalangeal, interphalangeal passive mobility
- Foot and ankle muscle strength
- Pulses: dorsalis pedis, posterior tibial
- Achilles' tendon reflex
- Special tests: Homans' sign (deep venous thrombosis), plantar fascia test (heel spur)

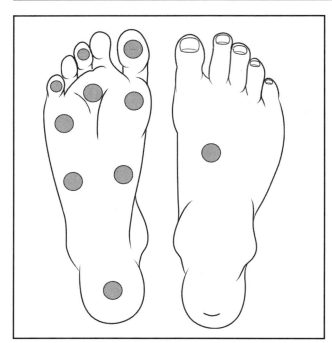

Figure 2-11. Tactile testing sites.

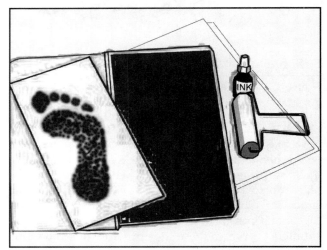

Figure 2-12. Harris mat and imprint.

ORTHOTIC INTERVENTIONS

Once the shoe has been selected it may be modified to improve the patient's comfort and function. Modifications may be internal (ie, placed within the shoe) or can be secured to the exterior of the shoe. In many instances, the same clinical disorder can be managed with either an internal or an external modification or a combination of modifications.

Inserts and Internal Modifications

The most common foot orthosis is an insert, which can be placed in many shoes assuming that the shoes were all made on the same last. An alternate foot ortho-

sis is an internal shoe modification, which is biomechanically identical to the insert but cannot be removed and transferred to another shoe. Neither the insert nor the internal shoe modification is visible when the shoe is worn. The advantage of the internal modification is that it guarantees that the patient wears the appropriate shoes when using the modification.

A three-quarter insert (Figure 2-13a) terminates just proximal to the metatarsal heads without crowding the forefoot. A full-length insert (Figure 2-13b) terminates at the distal end of the toe box, thereby preventing any slippage of the insert. The insert must fit snugly in the patient's shoe.

Heel spurs, Achilles' tendon contracture, and hindfoot malalignment are some hindfoot disorders that can be managed with internal heel modifications. Heel orthoses may benefit patients with leg length reduction, postural instability, and other disorders that originate outside the foot.

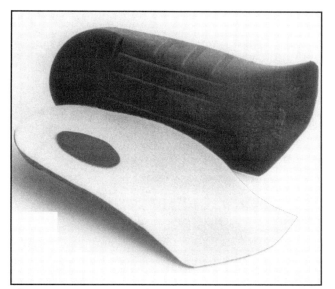

Figure 2-13a. Inserts—three-quarter length.

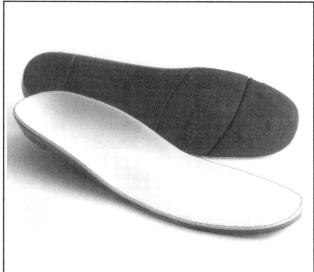

Figure 2-13b. Inserts—full length.

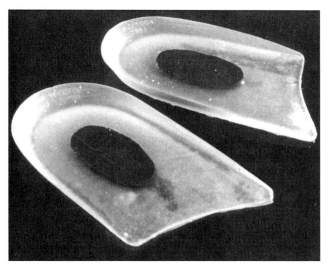

Figure 2-14. Tapered heel cushion.

Internal Heel Orthoses

These are often worn to reduce discomfort associated with heel spurs. A resilient, tapered cushion (Figure 2-14) absorbs shock at heel contact and transfers load to the forefoot. A heel orthosis with a wall, which surrounds the medial, posterior, and lateral portions of the anatomic heel, will reduce irritating sliding in the shoe. The cushion usually has a concave relief in the vicinity of the spur to minimize pressure.

Hind- and Midfoot Orthoses

Malalignment of the hind- and midfoot may result in either pes planus (pes valgus, pes planovalgus), in which the foot is abnormally pronated, or pes varus,

in which the foot is excessively supinated. The malalignment interferes with the smooth transition of weight from the heel to the toes during the stance phase of gait and may result in fatigue or pain. Reducing foot malalignment also diminishes patellofemoral pain[26] and discomfort from plantar fasciitis.

When the foot remains in a pronated posture during the stance phase, the patient is apt to experience hypermobility with consequent overuse of foot muscles, which results in fatigue. Foot orthoses for pes planus should apply an upward and laterally directed force to the talus and medially directed forces to the calcaneus and forefoot to counteract the abnormal foot alignment.

Inserts, whether mass-produced or custom-made, are formed of many different materials, ranging from rigid plastic to semirigid cork, molded leather and plastic to relatively resilient plastics.[27] The degree of optimal firmness is determined by the patient's weight, activity, and the extent of deformity. The greater the load on the foot, the firmer the orthosis.[28]

A medial heel wedge (post) within the shoe (Figure 2-15) may suffice, assuming that the shoe counter fits snugly. A shoe with a long medial counter is sometimes prescribed for children with flexible flat foot; the medial border of the counter terminates at the first metatarsophalangeal joint.

Another way to support the longitudinal arch in the presence of flexible deformity is an insert that has a medial vertical contour. Such orthoses are sometimes called arch supports. "Arch support" is a misleading term because normally one does not bear

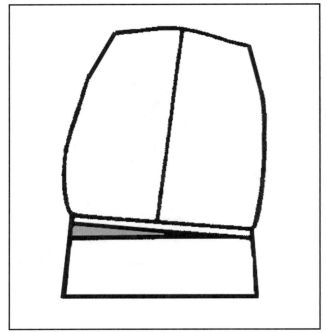

Figure 2-15. Medial heel wedge in a right shoe.

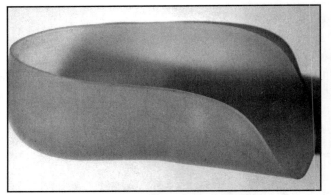

Figure 2-16. University of California Biomechanics Laboratory (UCBL) insert.

weight under the longitudinal arch. Weight should be borne under the calcaneal tuberosities in the hindfoot and the first and fifth metatarsal heads in the forefoot.

A particularly effective custom-made orthosis for flexible hyperpronation is the University of California Biomechanics Laboratory (UCBL) insert (Figure 2-16).[29] The orthosis holds the foot in the position of maximum correction. The UCBL improves foot alignment when the orthosis is worn[30] but does not appear to have a long-term effect. It is not intended for a rigid foot. The efficacy of foot orthoses on muscular activity and gait kinematics is debatable.[31-33]

An innovative shoe features a midsection fitted with a screw (Figure 2-17). One can raise or lower the height of the midsection to conform to the contour of the wearer's foot by adjusting the screw.

The foot that persists in hypersupination is relatively rigid and less able to absorb shock, particularly during early stance. The hypersupinated posture exists in pes cavus, in which the longitudinal arch is abnormally high. A resilient insert is beneficial, particularly if it has a total contact contour to increase pressure distribution.

Metatarsal Pad

A metatarsal pad (Figure 2-18) is used to reduce stress over the metatarsophalangeal joints. It has a convexity over the metatarsal shafts. The anterior margin of the pad terminates proximal to the metatarsal heads. Pads vary in shape, material, and resilience.[34]

For sesamoiditis, the insert has an anterior extension on the medial side. Toe deformities can be accommodated with a toe crest, which is a convex pad placed under the sulcus area of the toes, thereby increasing the bearing area to reduce pressure.[35]

Insoles

The contour and consistency of the sole have a marked effect on the wearer's comfort, stability, and walking ease. The insole influences pressure distribution and shock absorption. Flat inserts made of resilient plastic, such as closed-cell polyethylene foam, open-cell foam, viscoelastic polymer, silicone gel, or closed-cell neoprene sponge reduce high pressure concentrations when the foot is not markedly deformed. Resilient insoles are especially important for patients with diabetic neuropathy[36] and with poor balance.[37] Molded inserts conform to the plantar contour and are more effective in the presence of severe deformity. Some athletic shoes feature insoles with air chambers designed to absorb high impact.

External Modifications

Modification to the exterior of the shoe assures that suitable shoes will be worn and does not reduce space inside the shoe.[38-42] External modifications, however, are visible and may detract from the cosmetic appeal of the shoe.

Heel Modifications

These include a heel flare (Figure 2-19) (medial, lateral, or both) intended to stabilize the hindfoot. A resilient heel absorbs shock in the early stance phase of the gait cycle. It contributes to knee stability by causing the ground reaction force to pass closer to

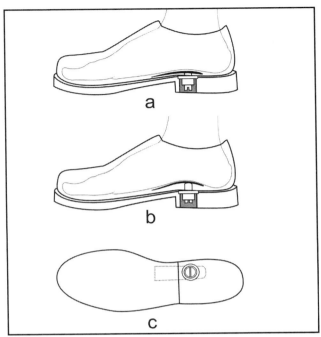

Figure 2-17. Screw-adjustable midsection. a. Low position. b. Elevated position. c. Plantar aspect.

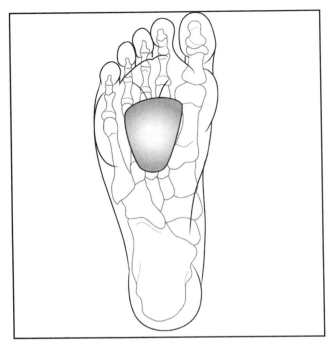

Figure 2-18. Metatarsal pad.

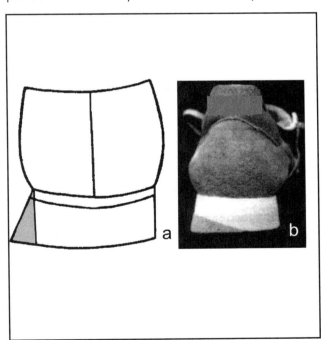

Figure 2-19. a. Medial heel flare in a right shoe. b. Resilient wedge in right heel.

the knee axis than is ordinarily the case. A heel with a posterior bevel also aids knee stability by the same biomechanical mechanism. The individual who wears a solid ankle AFO should wear a shoe with either a resilient heel or a beveled heel.

Medial and lateral heel wedges are external modifications that alter alignment of the entire foot. A resilient lateral heel wedge accommodates hindfoot varus without causing the midfoot to increase its pronation (see Figure 2-19).[43] The Thomas heel has its anterior border curved with a medial extension and a slight medial wedge.

Outsole

A resilient outsole attenuates differences in pressure concentration and absorbs shock.[44] Because a sponge rubber outsole is thicker than one made of leather, it shields the wearer from abrupt forces that would otherwise be imposed by irregularities in the walking surface. The rubber sole also improves traction between it and the pavement.

Rocker Bar

A rocker bar (Figure 2-20) on the sole has a plantar transverse convexity, which changes stance phase loading. The apex of the curve lies slightly posterior to the metatarsal heads. This configuration reduces time spent on the heads, thereby alleviating metatarsalgia.[45] Consequently, it enables the wearer to achieve late stance earlier than would be the case with a flat sole. The rocker is helpful for patients who have weak ankle plantar flexors. Propulsion during mid- and late stance, ordinarily achieved by triceps surae contraction, can be achieved by trunk momentum in the presence of the shorter sole length offered by the sole rocker. When used with patients who have diabetic neu-

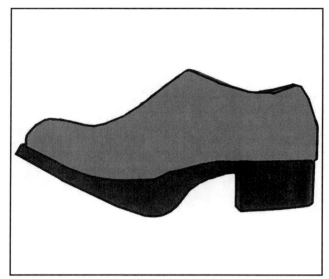

Figure 2-20. Rocker bar.

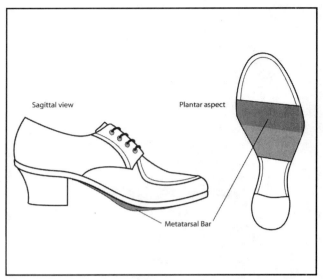

Figure 2-21. Metatarsal bar.

ropathy, the rocker sole resulted in earlier, diminished contraction of the dorsiflexors.[46] The rocker also diminishes the need for full ankle excursion, thus making the sole useful for the patient who has hind-foot pain or restriction of motion, or who wears an AFO that restricts dorsiflexion. Patients with limited metatarsophalangeal excursion can complete the stance phase more easily if the shoe has a rocker bar.

Metatarsal Bar

A metatarsal bar (Figure 2-21) is an external shoe modification that has a flat plantar surface that projects posteriorly from the forefoot. The bar lies transversely across the sole beneath the metatarsal shafts. It transfers load from the metatarsal heads to the shafts[47] and is indicated for patients complaining of metatarsalgia.

Heel and Sole Elevations

A heel elevation may be prescribed in the presence of pes equinus to foster weight-bearing on the heel when the patient stands and to enable the person to have heel and ankle rocker action during early stance. In case of leg-length discrepancy, the amount of lift should be determined empirically. A reasonable starting point is to note the height of lift blocks placed under the shorter leg to restore the pelvis to a level position. The lift will probably be 1/2 inch shorter than the stack of lift blocks. Part of the lift, usually 1/2 inch, can be located inside a low shoe, thus reducing the external lift. The external sole portion of the lift should be beveled to facilitate late stance and to prevent the toe from catching on the walking surface, which might cause the patient to trip.

For the patient with hemiparesis, a 1 cm heel and toe lift in the shoe on the nonparetic side facilitates paretic foot clearance during swing phase and improves weight-bearing symmetry during stance on the paretic side.[48]

FABRICATION OPTIONS

Orthoses, particularly FOs, can be mass-produced or custom-made. Regardless of mode of fabrication, the end result should fit the patient properly and should apply the desired forces.

Mass-produced FOs are made of felt, cork, rubber, and plastic foam. The clinician may perform minor modifications such as trimming or beveling a pad to suit a given patient. Over-the-counter inserts are less expensive than custom-made ones and are useful as a trial device and as a shock absorber.

A simple method for making resilient inserts involves cutting a rectangle of polyethylene foam slightly larger than the patient's foot. The clinician warms the plastic with a heat gun, hair dryer, or other source of dry heat, then places it on the floor. The patient stands on it with a stocking-covered foot. The material will be comfortably warm, but should not burn the skin because the cellular structure of the plastic dissipates heat. While the patient is bearing weight on the plastic, the clinician traces the contour of the foot on the plastic. After several minutes, the patient removes the foot from the plastic so that the clinician can cut the plastic along the traced outline of the foot. The resulting FO will be a resilient, total

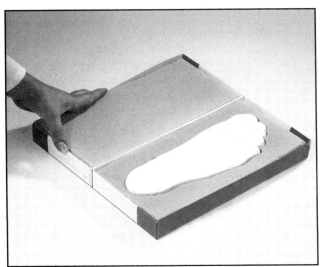

Figure 2-22. Impression casting foam box (reproduced with permission. © 2000 Birkenstock® Footprint Sandals, Inc. All rights reserved).

contact insert. Although the plastic will compress after a week or two of regular wear, the insert provides an excellent trial to determine the patient's response to a resilient insert. If the response is positive, then a more durable resilient insert should be provided to the patient.

Impression casts are usually made with a box of dry, closed-cell polystyrene foam (Figure 2-22). Usually, the patient is seated with the foot suspended. The clinician guides the foot to the top of the box, then presses down gently on the patient's thigh to achieve partial weight-bearing. After the impression is made, the clinician should lift the foot, heel first. The heel and forefoot imprints tend to be slightly wider and the arch slightly lower than in the unloaded foot. Once the impression is made, the clinician sends the box to a laboratory, where the impression is filled with liquid plaster and the insert made in a manner similar to that used with plaster casting. Foam casting is much cleaner and faster than plaster casting.

Plaster casting is another method for custom making an orthosis. The plantar aspect of the foot is wrapped in plaster, then the foot is guided in a subtalar neutral orientation into a full or partial weight-bearing position when a functional orthotic design is required. Sometimes the clinician applies pressure to the plaster-wrapped foot to emphasize loading on pressure-tolerant areas to relieve sensitive spots. The clinician can also alter the alignment of the foot, assuming articular mobility.[49] Regardless of the mode of casting, the resulting negative model is filled with liquid plaster to create a positive model. Plastics or other materials are then molded over the positive model to form the insert.

Another kind of insole is manufactured with a resin-filled compartment. Water injected into the compartment causes the resin to liquefy and expand. When the patient steps on the insole, it will conform to the plantar contour. If the clinician places a wedge beneath the foot, the insole will shape itself to the altered foot alignment.

In-shoe molding can also form a custom-made insert. Either the foot is wrapped with a thin layer of wet plaster and is encased in a thin plastic bag, or the shoe has a thermoforming plastic insert. With either method, the patient dons the shoe and stands in it, shaping the insert or plaster.

Some orthotists and pedorthists use computer-aided design (CAD) with or without computer-aided manufacture (CAM) to fabricate insoles.[50] The patient steps on a scanner, which records foot contour and loading pattern; the clinician can introduce various wedges to alter the loading pattern, usually so that it approximates a normative model. The CAM mill uses the CAD to shape materials into insoles.[51,52] Without the mill, the clinician uses the CAD-generated pattern as the basis for hand-fashioned insoles. Although effectiveness and patient satisfaction with CAD-CAM inserts are not significantly better than with hand-made devices, the cost is appreciably lower after the initial investment in the equipment has been amortized.

PEDIATRIC FOOT ORTHOSES

Two orthoses for the nonambulatory infant are the Denis Browne splint and the hinged shoe.

Denis Browne Splint

The Denis Browne splint (Figure 2-23) is a metal bar with attachments to the shoe soles. The device resists any tendency of the baby to adduct or internally rotate the hips. One version of the Denis Browne splint has a linkage that enables the child to flex and extend the legs at the hips. The splint is prescribed to maintain correction of talipes equinovarus in infants. The splint is also used to treat internal tibial torsion, although its efficacy has been challenged.[53] The effect is dissipated at the hip, knee, and ankle joints, rather than at the tibia.

Hinged Shoe

A shoe with a hinge at the midfoot can be used to treat metatarsus adductus. The shoe secures the fore-

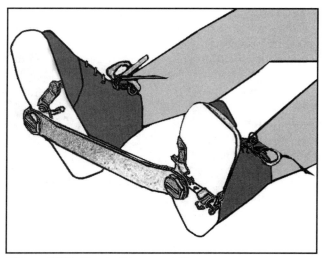

Figure 2-23. Denis Browne splint.

foot and hindfoot independently; the clinician adjusts the degree of rotation with a screw mechanism at the hinge.

GUIDELINES FOR PRESCRIPTION

The following are biomechanical guidelines for prescribing shoes and foot orthoses:

1. To reduce pressure on the heel
   a. Heel cushion
   b. Resilient insole
2. To stabilize the hindfoot
   a. Shoe with high, firm uppers
   b. Medial heel flare
   c. Lateral heel flare
   d. Bilateral heel flare
   e. Heel with resilient lateral wedge (to stabilize hindfoot varus)
3. To increase comfort in the presence of plantar fasciitis or patellofemoral discomfort
   a. Heel cushion or resilient heel
   b. Hind- and midfoot longitudinal support ("arch support")
4. To reduce flexible hyperpronation
   a. Medial heel wedge
   b. University of California Biomechanics Laboratory (UCBL) insert
   c. Hind- and midfoot longitudinal support ("arch support")
   d. Thomas heel
5. To accommodate fixed hyperpronation
   a. Shoe with long medial counter
6. To accommodate fixed hypersupination
   a. Resilient hind- and midfoot longitudinal support
7. To reduce pressure on the metatarsal heads
   a. Metatarsal pad
   b. Metatarsal bar
8. To reduce pressure on hammer toes or claw toes
   a. Shoe with a high toe box or extra depth
9. To reduce pressure on bunions
   a. Shoe with extra medial width; may be made on a bunion last
10. To reduce pressure on dorsal corns
    a. Shoe with a flexible upper, preferably moccasin-style
11. To stabilize the knee during early stance
    a. Resilient heel
    b. Beveled heel
12. To facilitate mid- and late stance
    a. Rocker bar

SUMMARY

Shoes have been part of people's wardrobes since prehistoric times. Rather than the term "orthopedic shoe," the perceptive clinician specifies the particular features of the shoe upper, heel, sole, and reinforcements that will benefit a given patient. Some individuals should be provided with special-purpose shoes, such as comfort or walking shoes, sandals, athletic shoes, or healing shoes featuring polyethylene foam uppers. Orthotic interventions include removable internal modifications known as inserts. These can be placed in many shoes, if all the shoes were made on the same last including the same heel height. Other orthoses are internal and external shoe modifications. Heel orthoses may contribute to standing stability or relieve the discomfort caused by heel pain. Hyperpronation control may be achieved with heel wedges, mass-produced inserts, or the custom-made UCBL insert. Inserts that contact the entire sole facilitate hypersupination control. Forefoot orthoses include metatarsal pads and bars, rocker soles, and resilient inserts. Heel and sole elevations may compensate for leg-length discrepancy. Some children are fitted with Denis Browne splints or hinged shoes for management of metatarsus adductus.

THOUGHT QUESTIONS

1. What is the relationship between midfoot pronation and the development of bunions? How can shoe selection and foot orthoses minimize or prevent bunions?

2. Explain the pathogenesis of plantar fasciitis and calcaneal heel spurs. How are foot orthoses used in the management of these conditions?

3. What shoe closure styles are suitable for a patient with hemiplegia and severe spasticity?

4. What shoe modification(s) should be suitable for a patient with forefoot adductus?

5. What are the benefits and drawbacks of a sandal for a patient with a healing diabetic ulcer?

6. What are the differences between a high heel in a woman's fashion shoe and a high heel prescribed for pes equinus?

7. Why is the sensory examination an important part of foot examination?

8. Explain how a metatarsal bar transfers load from the metatarsal heads to the metatarsal shafts. For which patient would this orthosis be appropriate?

REFERENCES

1. Boyd AG. Prehistoric shoe. *National Geographic.* 1999;195:45.

2. O'Keeffe L. *Shoes: A Celebration of Pumps, Sandals, Slippers, and More.* New York, NY: Workman Publishing; 1996.

3. Trasko M. *Heavenly Soles.* New York, NY: Abbeville Press; 1989.

4. Blakeslee TJ, Chan RJ. Chinese bound foot: a literature review and case report. *J Am Podiatr Med Assoc.* 1986;76:502-505.

5. Philipsen AB, Ellitsgaard N, Krogsgaard MR, Sonne-Holm S. Patient compliance and effect of orthopaedic shoes. *Prosthet Orthot Int.* 1999;23:59-62.

6. Roetzel B. *Gentlemen: A Timeless Fashion.* Cologne, Germany: Konemann; 1999:150-189.

7. Windle CM, Gregory SM, Dixon SJ. The shock attenuation characteristics of four different insoles when worn in a military boot during running and marching. *Gait Posture.* 1999;9:31-37.

8. Tooms RE, Griggin JW, Green S, Cagle K. Effect of viscoelastic insoles on pain. *Orthopedics.* 1987;10:1143-1146.

9. Corrigan JP, Moore DP, Stephens MM. Effect of heel height on forefoot loading. *Foot and Ankle.* 1993;14:148-152.

10. Gastwirth BW, O'Brien TD, Nelson RM, Manger DC, Kindig SA. An electrodynographic study of foot function in shoes of varying heel heights. *J Am Podiatr Med Assoc.* 1991;81:463-472.

11. Brecht JS, Chang MW, Price R, Lehmann J. Decreased balance performance in cowboy boots compared with tennis shoes. *Arch Phys Med Rehabil.* 1995;76:940-946.

12. Franklin ME, Chong RKY. Balance control during positive heel incline. *Neurology Report.* 1999;23:194.

13. Thompson FM, Coughlin MJ. The high price of high-fashion footwear. *J Bone Joint Surg [Am].* 1994;76:1586-1593.

14. de Lateur BJ, Giaconi RM, Questad K, et al. Footwear and posture: compensatory strategies for heel height. *Am J Phys Med Rehabil.* 1991;70:246-254.

15. Perry JE, Ulbrecht JS, Derr JA, Cavanagh PR. The use of running shoes to reduce plantar pressures in patients whom have diabetes. *J Bone Joint Surg [Am].* 1995;77:1819-1828.

16. Eng JJ, Pierrynowski MR. The effect of soft foot orthotics on three-dimensional lower-limb kinematics during walking and running. *Phys Ther.* 1994;74:836-844.

17. Cheskin MP. *The Complete Handbook of Athletic Footwear.* New York, NY: Fairchild Publications; 1987.

18. Johnson JA. Running shoes and orthoses: a practical approach. *Journal of Back and Musculoskeletal Rehabilitation.* 1996;6:71-80.

19. Kaye RA, Shereff MJ. Athletic footwear, modifications, and orthotic devices. In: Jahss MH, ed. *Disorders of the Foot and Ankle: Medical and Surgical Management.* 2nd ed. Philadelphia, Pa: WB Saunders; 1991:2910-2922.

20. Edelstein JE. If the shoe fits: footwear considerations for the elderly. *Physical and Occupational Therapy in Geriatrics.* 1987;5:1-16.

21. Lord M, Hosein R. Pressure redistribution by molded inserts in diabetic footwear: a pilot study. *J Rehabil Res Dev.* 1994;31:214-221.

22. Mueller MJ, Strube MJ. Therapeutic footwear: enhanced function in people with diabetes and transmetatarsal amputation. *Arch Phys Med Rehabil.* 1997;78:951-956.

23. Jahss MH. *Disorders of the Foot and Ankle: Medical and Surgical Management.* 2nd ed. Philadelphia, Pa: WB Saunders; 1991.

24. Pham H, Armstrong DG, Harvey C, Harkless LB, Giurini JM, Veves A. Screening techniques to identify people at high risk for diabetic foot ulceration: a prospective multicenter trial. *Diabetes Care.* 2000;23:606-611.

25. Cavanagh PR, Hewitt FG, Perry JE. In-shoe pressure measurement: a review. *Foot.* 1992;2:185-195.

26. Pitman D, Jack D. A clinical investigation to determine the effectiveness of biomechanical foot orthoses as initial treatment for patellofemoral pain syndrome. *Journal of Prosthetics and Orthotics.* 2000;12:110-116.

27. Johanson MA, Donatelli R, Wooden MJ, Andrew PD, Cummings GS. Effects of three different posting methods on controlling abnormal subtalar pronation. *Phys Ther.* 1994;74:149-161.

28. Brown GP, Donatelli R, Catlin PA, Wooden MJ. The effect of two types of foot orthoses on rearfoot mechanics. *J Orthop Sports Phys Ther.* 1995;21:258-267.

29. Henderson WH, Campbell JW. UCBL shoe insert—casting and fabrication. *Bulletin of Prosthetics Research.* 1969;Spring:215-235.

30. Mereday C, Dolan CME, Lusskin R. Evaluation of the University of California Biomechanics Laboratory shoe insert in "flexible pes planus." *Clin Orthop.* 1972;82:45-51.

31. Leung AKL, Mak AFT, Evans JH. Biomechanical gait evaluation of the immediate effect of orthotic treatment for flexible flat foot. *Prosthet Orthot Int.* 1998;22:25-34.

32. Staheli L, Chew DE, Corbett M. The longitudinal arch: a survey of eight hundred eighty-two feet in normal children and adults. *J Bone Joint Surg [Am].* 1987;69:426-428.

33. Tomaro J, Burdett RG. The effects of foot orthotics on the EMG activity of selected leg muscles during gait. *J Orthop Sports Phys Ther.* 1993;18:532-536.

34. Bordelon RL. *Surgical and Conservative Foot Care: A Unified Approach to Principles and Practice.* Thorofare, NJ: SLACK Incorporated; 1988.

35. Cailliet R. *Foot and Ankle Pain.* 3rd ed. Philadelphia, Pa: FA Davis Company; 1997.

36. Birke JA, Foto JG, Pfiefer LA. Effect of orthosis material hardness on walking pressure in high-risk diabetes patients. *Journal of Prosthetics and Orthotics.* 1999;11:43-46.

37. Robbins S, Gouw GI, McClaran J. Shoe sole thickness and hardness influence balance in older men. *J Am Geriatr Soc.* 1992;40:1089-1094.

38. Gould N. Shoes and shoe modifications. In: Jahss MH, ed. *Disorders of the Foot and Ankle: Medical and Surgical Management.* 2nd ed. Philadelphia, Pa: WB Saunders; 1991:2879-2909.

39. Janisse DJ, Wertsch JJ, Del Toro DR. Foot orthoses and prescription shoes. In: Redford JB, Basmajian JV, Trautman P, eds. *Orthotics: Clinical Practice and Rehabilitation Technology.* New York, NY: Churchill Livingstone; 1995:55-70.

40. Reiley MA. *Guidelines for Prescribing Foot Orthotics.* Thorofare, NJ: SLACK Incorporated; 1995.

41. Schwartz RS. Foot orthoses and materials. In: Jahss MH, ed. *Disorders of the Foot and Ankle: Medical and Surgical Management.* 2nd ed. Philadelphia, Pa: WB Saunders; 1991:2866-2878.

42. Wu KK. *Foot Orthoses: Principles and Clinical Applications.* Baltimore, Md: Williams & Wilkins; 1990.

43. Glancy J. *Orthotic Recommendations: Management of Functional Forefoot Drop.* Indianapolis, Ind: John Glancy; 2000.

44. Alexander IJ, Chao EYS, Johnson KA. The assessment of dynamic foot-to-ground contact forces and plantar pressure distribution: a review of the evolution of current techniques and clinical applications. *Foot and Ankle.* 1990;11:152-167.

45. Posema K, Burm PET, Zande ME, Limbeek J. Primary metatarsalgia: the influence of a custom moulded insole and a rockerbar on plantar pressure. *Prosthet Orthot Int.* 1998;22:35-44.

46. Harris G, Klein J, Janisse D, et al. Effect of rocker-soles on lower extremity dynamic EMG patterns [abstract]. *Gait Posture.* 2000;11:158.

47. Rubin G, Staros A. Orthotic and prosthetic management of foot disorders. In: Jahss MH, ed. *Disorders of the Foot and Ankle: Medical and Surgical Management.* 2nd ed. Philadelphia, Pa: WB Saunders; 1991:2808-2833.

48. Chaudhuri S, Aruin AS. The effect of shoe lifts on static and dynamic postural control in individuals with hemiparesis. *Arch Phys Med Rehabil.* 2000;81:1498-1503.

49. Cummings GS, Higbie EJ. A weight-bearing method for determining forefoot posting for orthotic fabrication. *Physiother Res Int.* 1997;2:42-50.

50. Janisse DJ. Orthoses, shoewear, and shoe modifications. In: Myerson MS, ed. *Foot and Ankle Disorders.* Philadelphia, Pa: WB Saunders Company; 2000:195-212.

51. Davis FM. In-office computerized fabrication of custom foot supports: the AMFIT system. *Clin Podiatr Med Surg.* 1993;10:393-401.

52. Tait JR, Redford JB, Johnson JC. Evaluation of AMFIT (Computer Generated Soft Foot Orthoses) in a veteran population. *Arch Phys Med Rehabil.* 1996;77:986. Abstract.

53. Gold JT. Orthotic management and rehabilitation of the foot and ankle in the neurologically impaired child. In: Jahss MH, ed. *Disorders of the Foot and Ankle: Medical and Surgical Management.* 2nd ed. Philadelphia, Pa: WB Saunders; 1991:2775-2796.

RECOMMENDED READING

1. Arnadottir SA, Mercer VS. Effects of footwear on measurements of balance and gait in women between the ages of 65 and 93 years. *Phys Ther.* 2000;80:17-27.

2. Cornwall MW, McPoil TG. Plantar fasciitis: etiology and treatment. *J Orthop Sports Phys Ther.* 1999;29:756-760.

3. Donatelli RA. *The Biomechanics of the Foot and Ankle.* 2nd ed. Philadelphia, Pa: FA Davis Company; 1996.

4. Mueller MJ. Application of plantar pressure assessment in footwear and insert design. *J Orthop Sports Phys Ther.* 1999;29:747-755.

5. Myerson MS. *Foot and Ankle Disorders*. Philadelphia, Pa: WB Saunders Company; 2000.

6. Nawoczenski DA. Nonoperative and operative intervention for hallux rigidus. *J Orthop Sports Phys Ther.* 1999;29:727-735.

7. Shrader JA. Nonsurgical management of the foot and ankle affected by rheumatoid arthritis. *J Orthop Sports Phys Ther.* 1999;29:703-717.

8. Sinacore DR, Withrington NC. Recognition and management of acute neuropathic (Charcot) arthropathies of the foot and ankle. *J Orthop Sports Phys Ther.* 1999;29:736-746.

CASE STUDIES

For the following cases, select an appropriate orthosis, establish long- and short-term treatment goals, and develop a treatment plan.

- BK is a 23-year-old waitress who runs 10 miles a week. She has developed shin splints in both legs and has started to complain recently of low back pain. She stands with both knees hyperextended, her pelvis is tilted anteriorly, and she has an increased lumbar lordosis. What is an appropriate foot orthosis?

- JT is a 35-year-old appliance salesman who plays handball 5 days a week. He complains of chronic blisters and calluses on his feet and medial knee pain bilaterally. He has severe midfoot hyperpronation bilaterally and moderate bunion deformities. What is an appropriate foot orthosis?

- RC is a 45-year-old secretary who has had chronic low back pain with left-sided sciatica for the past 20 years. She has consulted many health care professionals and has tried multiple interventions. Treatments usually are effective in the short-term, but the pain returns after sev-

eral weeks. She has decided to see a physical therapist, who noted pelvic obliquity with the right hip lower than the left. RC has positive sacroiliac tests on the left. The left lower extremity is 1 inch longer than the right. What is the probable cause of her low back pain? What is an appropriate foot orthosis?

- FP is a 32-year-old machinist with insulin-dependent diabetes. Sensation is intact with no open areas on the feet. On both feet, calluses are present on the medial aspect of the great toe; on the plantar aspect of metatarsal heads I, II, and III; and on the lateral aspect of the heel. He hyperpronates when walking. What is an appropriate foot orthosis?

- AD is a 47-year-old bus driver with painful plantar fasciitis on her left foot. When she is not working, she spends most of her time watching television. She is 40 pounds overweight. Both feet are high-arched. She walks on the lateral border of her left foot. What is an appropriate foot orthosis?

POINT/COUNTERPOINT

A 55-year-old department store buyer has worn dress shoes with 3-inch heels for the past 30 years. She complains of forefoot pain, particularly under the second and third metatarsal heads, bilaterally. She has moderate bunions, several ingrown toenails, hammer toes, edema, and ligamentous laxity. She is 15 pounds overweight. Her shoes are at least a half size too short and too narrow.

JOAN SAYS

JAN SAYS

Shoe Selection

Because her job requires fashionable dress, I recommend attractive shoes with 2-inch heels, preferably lower. Shoes should have a curved, rather than pointed, toe box. The toe box should be spacious enough to accommodate her hammer toes. The shoes should be adequately long and wide. The pedorthist may have to stretch the leather in the vicinity of the bunion. Otherwise, a shoe that is wide enough to accommodate the bunion will be excessively roomy in the back, creating irritation during late stance.

I agree that she will be more accepting of fashionable shoes. I would compromise with a low-heeled pump with an upper that extends midway on the dorsum of the foot to minimize pressure on the metatarsal heads. The shoe should have a flattened heel pitch and sturdy counter to control hyperpronation.

Foot Orthosis

Full-length resilient insert with metatarsal pad for each shoe to transfer stress from the metatarsal heads to the metatarsal shafts. The insert will absorb shock.

If the bunion is manually reducible, improve balance between the calcaneus and metatarsal heads. Otherwise, provide a UCBL insert for hindfoot control, making certain that the insert fits snugly in her shoe. A heel cushion will absorb shock at initial contact.

Long-Term Goals

Of particular importance is her comfort during the workday. As a department store buyer, this woman has to walk in wholesalers' showrooms and display the new selections for the sales staff at the department store.

To increase her walking comfort, I would like to reduce her bunions, if possible, as well as eliminate pain under each forefoot.

Short-Term Goals

In addition to guiding her shoe selection and obtaining a pair of resilient inserts, I would teach her how to increase her forefoot mobility, especially at metatarsophalangeal and interphalangeal joints.

I would help her to identify stylish, yet comfortable shoes. I would encourage her to use the orthosis until the plantar fascia, midfoot, and transverse tarsal capsules tighten enough to maintain improved foot posture with reduction in pain.

| JOAN SAYS | JAN SAYS |

Physical Therapy Plans

- Tepid foot bath to prepare for mobility exercises
- Resistive foot exercise with a Turkish towel; emphasize strengthening the toe extensors and abductors

- Foot bath
- Deep tissue massage
- Passive foot mobilization to reduce bunions, followed by active range of motion exercise to maintain functional range of motion

Chapter 3

Ankle-Foot Orthoses

"Man's feet are his fate."
Babylonian Talmud, Sukkah 53a

Ankle-foot orthoses (AFOs) control the alignment and motion of the foot and ankle and thereby affect the entire body. They are less expensive, more cosmetically acceptable, and more energy efficient than more extensive bracing. In addition, they may enable the patient to achieve the same functional goals as would be possible with KAFOs and higher orthoses.

PLASTIC ANKLE-FOOT ORTHOSES

For individuals who need ankle control, AFOs made of plastic, such as polypropylene, are the standard orthosis. They are lightweight and require minimal maintenance. Usually, the posterior aspect of the AFO (calf shell) contacts the back of the leg; the calf shell is secured anteriorly with a hook-and-pile strap. The plantar aspect (shoe insert) contacts the sole of the foot. The shoe is an integral part of this orthotic system.[1] The plastic AFO includes a shoe insert, which is made for a shoe of a specific heel height. If the shoe heel is too high, the wearer's knee will be unstable. If the heel is too low, the wearer may develop pain in the popliteal fossa.

An AFO applies a three-point pressure system to the limb. The correcting, anteriorly directed force (A_1) is located at the calf shell and is opposed by a distal, posteriorly directed force (P) on the dorsum of the foot from the shoe and a distal, superiorly directed force (A_2) supplied by the shoe sole and insert[2] (Figure 3-1).

The orthotist makes the AFO by molding plastic on a plaster model of the patient's lower leg, drawing a line on the plastic to indicate where the plastic will be cut. This line is called a trimline (Figure 3-2) and will determine how much control the orthosis will apply. Trimlines that lie anterior to the malleoli produce a more rigid orthosis. Those cut posterior to the malleoli are found on less rigid appliances. The control offered by the orthosis also depends on the type and rigidity of the plastic.

Posterior Leaf Spring

For patients who have weak dorsiflexors, an AFO posterior leaf spring (AFO-PLS) (Figure 3-3) is quite effective in preventing toe drag during swing phase and foot slap during loading response. The PLS has a shoe insert secured to the foot by the shoe upper. The insert is continuous with a vertical strip forming the calf shell, which is trimmed posterior to the malleoli. The proximal aspect of the calf shell is

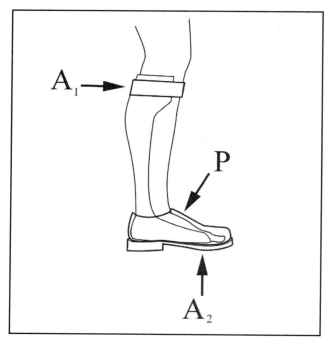

Figure 3-1. Three-point force system in an AFO.

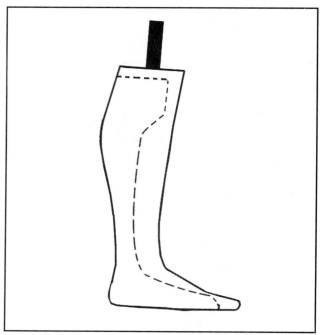

Figure 3-2. Trimline drawn on a plaster model.

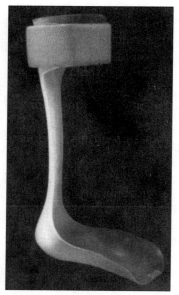

Figure 3-3. Ankle-foot orthosis—posterior leaf spring.

and body weight is transferred onto the opposite limb during preswing, the AFO allows a few degrees of plantar flexion. When off-loaded during the swing phase, the PLS functions as a spring to bring the ankle back to neutral position, preventing toe drag.[3]

The PLS has no mechanical ankle joint. Ankle motion is permitted by the deformation and recoil of the vertical plastic strip. Because this arrangement places the center of rotation of the orthosis considerably behind the center of rotation of the talocrural joint, pistoning of the orthosis may occur. The patient must wear a sock between the skin and the plastic to protect the skin from abrasion. For those who need more control, the plastic can be corrugated (Figure 3-4). When a material is creased, it resists right-angle deformation. Creasing increases the rigidity of the appliance without adding weight. A distal calf shell with an "X" design eliminates pressure over the Achilles' tendon.

The PLS offers minimal resistance to mediolateral and transverse rotation of the ankle and foot.

Spiral AFO

A spiral AFO encircles the leg (Figures 3-5a and 3-5b). The appliance consists of a shoe insert and a narrow proximal strip that is molded into a 360-degree spiral. The spiral arises from the medial aspect of the insert, wraps around the leg, and terminates near the medial tibial condyle. The semirigid plastic uncurls slightly during early stance as the limb accepts

trimmed below the head of the fibula and the popliteal fossa. An anterior strap secures the orthosis to the proximal leg.

This design permits the plastic to bend and recoil slightly through the gait cycle. The PLS allows ankle plantarflexion when the patient transfers body weight onto the braced stance limb during loading response. As the leg progresses over the fixed foot during midstance, the plastic bends to enable slight ankle dorsiflexion. As the foot rises off the ground

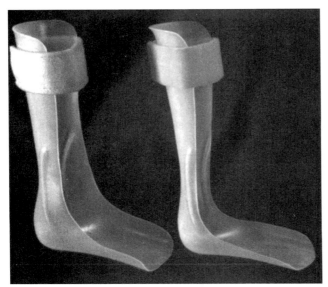

Figure 3-4. AFOs with corrugations.

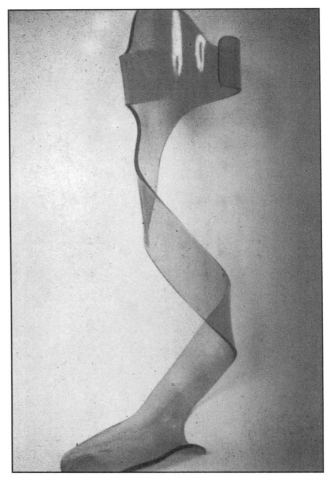

Figure 3-5a. Spiral AFO—orthosis.

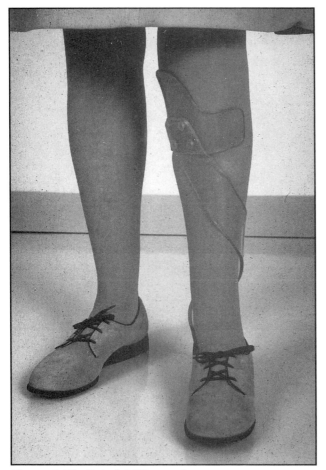

Figure 3-5b. Spiral AFO—on leg.

weight, permitting some ankle plantarflexion. The spiral returns to its original shape as the ankle comes to neutral position in midstance. From midstance through terminal stance, the spiral compresses like a coiled spring as the ankle dorsiflexes. With heel rise in preswing, the stance limb is off-loaded, allowing the spiral to uncoil slightly to assist in plantar flexion. During the swing phase, the spiral returns to its original shape to support the forefoot, thereby preventing toe drag. The spiral AFO is lightweight, streamlined, and fastener-free, making it relatively easy to don. Because it must fit snugly and cannot be adjusted by the wearer, the spiral AFO is contraindicated in the presence of marked edema. The hemispiral (Figures 3-6a and 3-6b), which arises from the lateral aspect of the shoe insert, wraps 180 degrees and terminates near the medial tibial condyle, providing more rigid control of pes varus.[4]

Both the spiral and hemispiral AFOs are contraindicated for patients with marked spasticity. Individuals with severe cognitive problems or apraxia will need assistance in donning these orthoses.

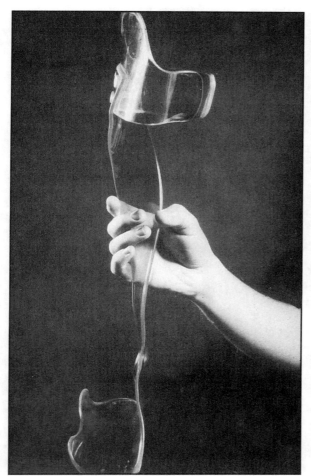

Figure 3-6a. Hemispiral AFO—orthosis.

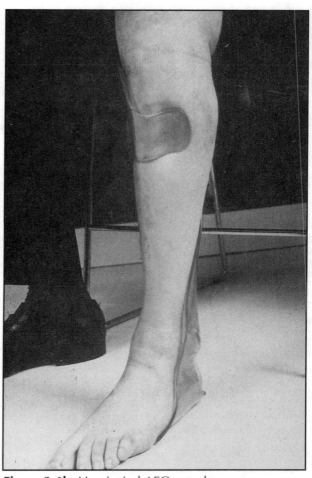

Figure 3-6b. Hemispiral AFO—on leg.

Solid Ankle Designs

With trimlines anterior to the malleoli (Figure 3-7), the solid ankle AFO (AFO-SA) surrounds most of the ankle, preventing ankle and hindfoot movement. The SA maintains the ankle-foot alignment in the position in which the patient's limb was cast. Restricting ankle and foot motion usually serves to suppress spasticity for patients with upper motor neurological deficits. The SA does not let the ankle plantarflex or the foot invert as part of the extensor synergy during weight-bearing and it guards against sudden dorsiflexion, which might elicit clonus. The SA is also indicated to control a flaccid foot and ankle.

The SA will resist a hyperextended knee such as may be present in the patient who compensates for quadriceps weakness by forcing the knee to yield into hyperextension. The proximal portion of the calf shell provides an anteriorly directed force near the knee to restrain hyperextension, and the distal portion of the calf shell blocks plantar- and dorsiflexion.

The benefits of the SA must be weighed against its drawbacks. The SA alters the ankle's action in gait. During loading response, the foot normally plantarflexes to achieve foot flat without undue knee flexion. The SA, however, maintains a rigid foot and ankle alignment. Consequently, the braced foot cannot be lowered gently to the ground to achieve foot flat.[5] A SA worn with a shoe having a heel that compresses readily during early stance reduces the flexion moment at the knee (Figure 3-8).

In midstance, the SA inhibits the normal ankle rocker mechanism. As body weight passes over the foot, the orthosis restricts the usual dorsiflexion moment at the ankle. Instead, body weight progresses over a rigid foot and ankle, placing more flexion stress on the knee and hip. Unless the quadriceps are very strong, rapid progression of the leg over the immobile foot can destabilize the knee. Many patients avoid the risk of knee collapse by shortening their step length and contacting the ground with a flat foot, walking more slowly, or by externally rotat-

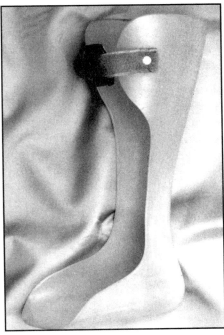

Figure 3-7. Solid ankle ankle-foot orthosis.

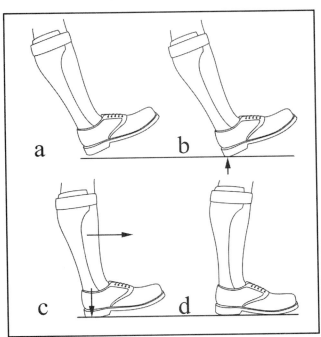

Figure 3-8. Biomechanics of an AFO-SA with resilient heel: a. end of swing phase in preparation for heel strike; b. at heel strike ground reaction force pushes up on heel; c. resilient heel compresses in response to ground forces permitting lower leg to rotate forward in a controlled manner; d. sole achieves full floor contact at midstance.

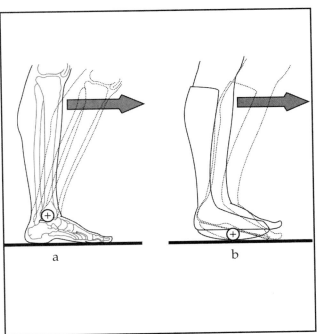

Figure 3-9. Biomechanics of an AFO-SA with rocker sole. + indicates axis of rotation. a. Unbraced leg. b. Leg with AFO-SA.

ing the hip to contact the ground on the lateral aspect of the foot. In late stance, the dorsiflexion moment increases. All of these changes serve to destabilize the knee. A rocker sole facilitates leg advancement during midstance and terminal stance (Figure 3-9).

Because it lacks an ankle joint, the AFO-SA tends to slide up and down slightly on the leg during the stance phase. Consequently, the patient should wear a high sock to shield the skin from abrasion. Wearers may compensate for the piston-like sliding by walking with shorter steps and externally rotating the braced leg.

The calf shell can be trimmed to extend just above the malleoli to provide slight mobility around the ankle. The supramalleolar design functions like a sturdy boot (Figure 3-10), supporting the ankle in all planes while permitting slight talocrural motion. As is the case with the SA, the supramalleolar AFO has no moving parts, so it is durable and lightweight.

Hinged AFOs

To enable ankle motion while maintaining more mediolateral control than the PLS affords, some AFOs include ankle joints (Figure 3-11). Plastic joints are generally lighter in weight, are more streamlined, require less maintenance, but are less durable than metal joints. They are used more frequently in children's orthoses because young patients weigh less and generate lower forces.

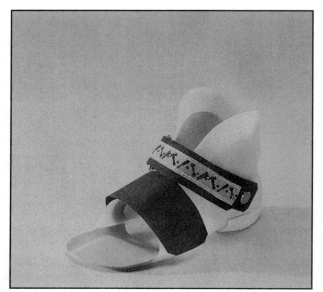

Figure 3-10. Supramalleolar AFO.

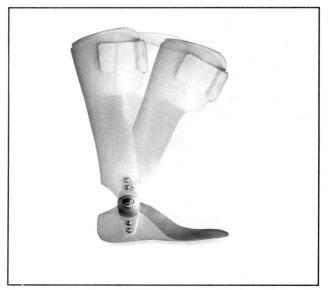

Figure 3-11. Hinged ankle joint (Camber Axis Hinge® reproduced with permission of Becker Orthopedic).

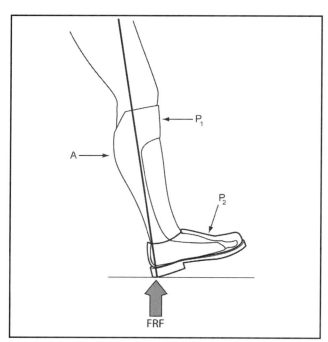

Figure 3-12. Biomechanics of an AFO-SA with an anterior band.

Hinges are manufactured to permit unrestricted motion (sometimes called free motion) or variable plantar flexion or dorsiflexion control. A posterior stop resists plantar flexion, while an anterior stop blocks dorsiflexion. The design of a specific joint and the orientation of the orthotic trimlines[6] affect the wearer's function. Hinges on plastic AFOs should be aligned with the malleoli and with the frontal plane.

Malalignment can result in excessive pistoning motion or abnormal rotation of the leg during weight-bearing.

Hinged orthoses present disadvantages for some patients. Motion at the ankle may stimulate increased tone or clonus in those individuals who have certain neuropathies. Hinged AFOs are heavier, less durable, and bulkier than the SA designs.

AFO-SA with an Anterior Band

For patients with quadriceps weakness who do not exhibit genu recurvatum with extensor spasticity, knee flexion control can be achieved with an AFO-SA with an anterior band. This appliance, sometimes called a floor reaction orthosis, has a semirigid band in place of the customary anterior strap. The anterior band provides a posteriorly directed force that stabilizes the knee in early stance by preventing the ground reaction force vector from passing too far behind the knee joint (Figure 3-12).

During midstance, the anterior band continues to stabilize the knee, while the calf shell provides mediolateral and rotational control at the distal leg and ankle. This arrangement controls the knee, yet it allows knee flexion during late stance and swing phase. A rocker shoe sole will maintain forward momentum during the stance phase. The AFO-SA with the anterior band is ineffective in controlling the knee that has a flexion contracture.

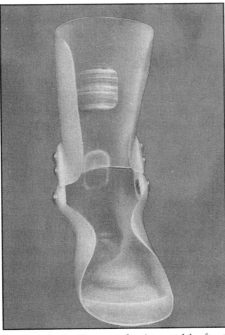

Figure 3-13. Tone-reducing ankle-foot orthosis.

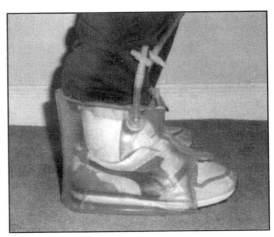

Figure 3-14. Air splint.

Tone-Reducing and Tone-Inhibiting AFOs

Tone-reducing AFOs (TRAFOs) and tone-inhibiting AFOs (TIAFOs) reduce tone in patients with neurological lesions associated with hypertonicity.[7,8] The TRAFO (Figure 3-13) calf shell extends from midcalf to the shoe insert. The insert has a distal wedge under the metatarsal heads to abduct the toes. A strap over the dorsum of the foot or a snug shoe closure controls the midfoot and holds the hindfoot in the best attainable alignment. This positioning of the foot and ankle prevents the patient from activating the extensor synergy during stance phase. When the ankle dorsiflexes during midstance and terminal stance, the leg pulls away from the shell. During presswing as the ankle plantar flexes, the leg presses against the shell, giving proprioceptive and tactile input to stimulate ankle dorsiflexion and minimize toe drag during swing. The relatively rigid posterior portion of the orthosis also contributes to swing phase foot control.

TIAFOs, such as air splints (Figure 3-14), provide another way of inhibiting spastic patterns.[9,10] The inflatable plastic splint inhibits spastic flexion and extension patterns. Both tone-inhibiting casts and TIAFOs provide the following:

1. Prolonged stretch of the ankle plantar flexors and long toe flexors
2. Constant pressure on the tendons of the long toe flexors
3. Inhibition of reflexes induced by tactile stimulation
4. Weight-bearing in proper alignment to influence proprioceptors through joint compression
5. Altered muscle length resulting in change in resistance to passive stretch
6. Improved recruitment and sequencing of muscle activity[8]

Flanged AFOs

To control excessive supination or pronation, the AFO may have a flange on the calf shell. The flange is padded and positioned proximal to the ankle joint to resist the undesired motion. A lateral flange controls excessive supination, and a medial flange (Figure 3-15) resists excessive pronation.

LEATHER-METAL ANKLE-FOOT ORTHOSES

Before the advent of polypropylene and similar plastics, orthoses were made of steel or aluminum with leather accessories. Leather-metal AFOs include a steel fixture that is attached to the shoe, ankle joints, uprights, and a calf band with a closure strap (Figure 3-16). Both the leather-metal and the plastic AFOs provide a modular approach to orthotic management by allowing multiple options in components. When compared with the plastic AFOs, the leather-metal designs provide better accommodation for uncontrolled edema and dermatitis. Shoes are

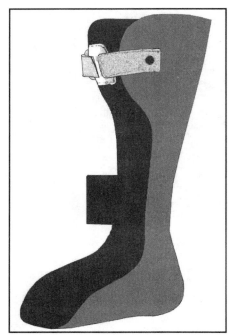

Figure 3-15. Left AFO with medial flange.

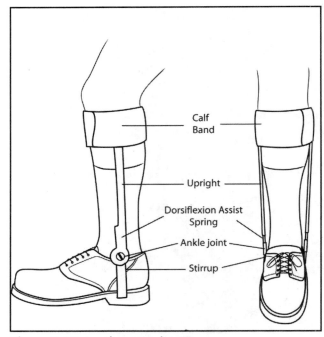

Figure 3-16. Leather-metal AFO.

riveted to the stirrups, thus ensuring that the AFO will be worn with the appropriate footwear. The secure attachment also increases the likelihood of third-party reimbursement for the shoes.

Negative aspects of the leather-metal design focus on the longer time needed for donning the orthosis, difficulty changing footwear, poorer appearance, and higher energy expenditure. The disparity between plastic and leather-metal orthoses is diminishing as the demand for lighter, more cosmetic, and energy-effective materials is resulting in steel and aluminum occasionally being replaced by titanium, fiberglass, and composites; however, orthoses made of newer materials are more difficult to shape and modify and are appreciably more expensive. Leather straps and pads are being replaced by Dacron webbing (Pel Supply Company, Cleveland, Ohio), hook-and-pile tape, and other synthetic materials. In spite of the introduction of newer materials, the basic leather-metal designs remain unchanged.

Stirrups and Calipers

The distal component of the leather-metal AFO is either a stirrup or a caliper. Stirrups are manufactured in solid and split models. A solid stirrup is a U-shaped piece of steel (Figure 3-17) that is riveted to the sole and steel shank of a sturdy shoe at a point corresponding to the anterior aspect of the calcaneus.

Bilateral or unilateral uprights rise from the side portions of the stirrup and are bent so that the mechanical ankle joint of the orthosis is aligned with the anatomical ankle joint.

The split stirrup has three pieces: a steel plate with a transverse slot and two flat L-shaped uprights that fit into the slot (Figure 3-18). The plate is riveted to the sole and shank of the shoe. Donning is facilitated because the patient can detach the shoe from the proximal portions of the orthosis. To attach the uprights to the shoe, the wearer inserts the distal portion of each upright into its respective slot. The individual can change shoes provided that each shoe is equipped with a plate. The split stirrup option is heavier, thicker, and less durable than the solid stirrup and is contraindicated for patients who have severe torsional movements. An abrupt rotatory thrust can cause the distal aspect of the upright to withdraw from the slot. As a result, the orthosis will no longer be able to provide ankle support for the wearer.

An alternative to the split stirrup is the caliper. It consists of a steel tube placed in the shoe's heel. Round L-shaped uprights are inserted into the medial and lateral ends of the tube. Benefits of the caliper design include ease in donning and doffing and the relatively low cost. The major drawback of this design is that the orthotic joint axis is appreciably

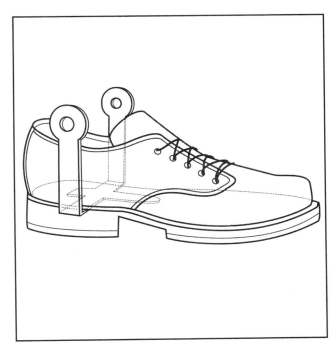

Figure 3-17. Solid stirrup.

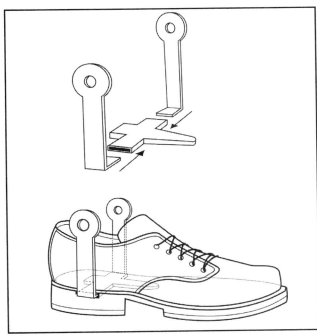

Figure 3-18. Split stirrup.

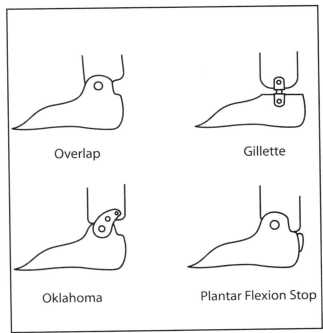

Figure 3-19. Ankle joints attached to plastic shoe inserts.

distal to the anatomical axis. This arrangement results in the proximal portion of the AFO sliding up and down on the calf, causing skin irritation. The extent of pistoning is proportional to the motion occurring at the anatomical ankle joint.

Ankle Joints

To permit talocrural motion, orthoses usually have plastic or steel ankle joints. The sturdier metal joints are indicated for adults and active children. Ankle joints can be attached to metal stirrups and to plastic shoe inserts (Figure 3-19). Steel ankle joints have a single axis that can provide control for plantar flexion, dorsiflexion, or both motions. The stirrup, in combination with the shoe and uprights, provides mediolateral and rotational control. If only mediolateral and rotational control is required, the orthosis can have a free motion joint, which offers no resistance to sagittal plane motion.

Ankle Stops

Mechanical ankle joints ordinarily have stops to restrict ankle motion to a predetermined range. A plantar flexion stop has a projection on the posterior section within the joint that limits plantar flexion (Figure 3-20). A dorsiflexion stop has an anterior projection that limits dorsiflexion (Figure 3-21). A limited-motion stop has projections on both the anterior and posterior sections of the joint, thus restricting motion in both directions (Figure 3-22).

Ankle Assists

As the name implies, some mechanisms assist ankle motion by substituting for weak or paralyzed

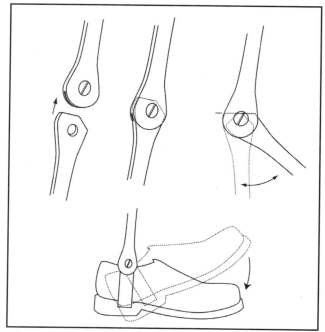

Figure 3-20. Plantar flexion stop.

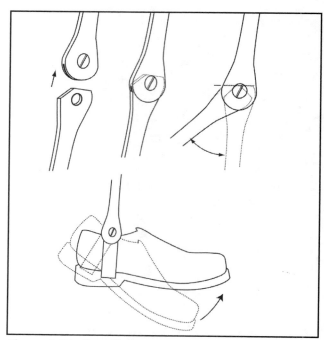

Figure 3-21. Dorsiflexion stop.

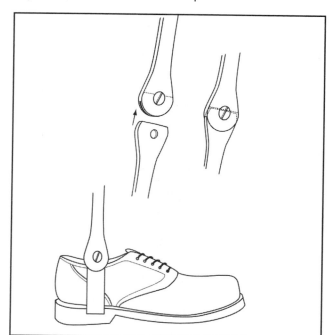

Figure 3-22. Limited-motion stop.

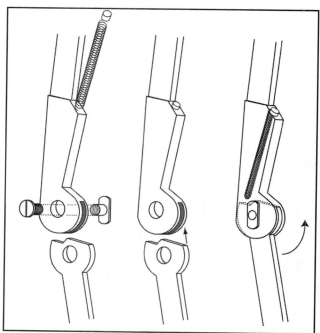

Figure 3-23. Dorsiflexion assist.

muscles. A dorsiflexion assist (Figure 3-23) consists of a spring inside the mechanical ankle joint. A top screw maintains the desired compression of the coil. The spring compresses during weight acceptance when the ankle plantarflexes. The spring recoils to assist dorsiflexion when load is removed from the limb. The action of the spring controls plantar flexion during loading response and preswing, as well as prevents toe drag during swing phase. Because the forces involved are relatively small, a dorsiflexion spring assist need only be strong enough to counteract the weight of the foot and the shoe.

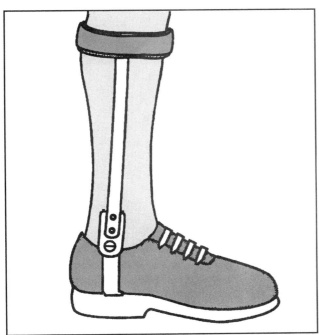

Figure 3-24. Leather-metal AFO with bichannel adjustable ankle lock (BiCAAL) joint.

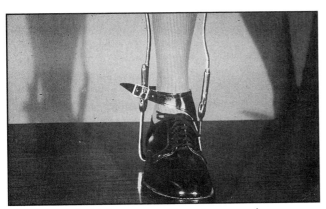

Figure 3-25b. Valgus correction strap—on leg.

No spring can substitute for the action of the plantar flexor muscles yet be suitably small. Instead, clinicians sometimes use the bichannel adjustable ankle lock (BiCAAL) joint, which has anterior and posterior springs (Figure 3-24). Once the desired ankle alignment is achieved, the top screws are tightened so that the joint can resist all sagittal motion. The BiCAAL joint permits adjusting the alignment of the upright to suit the body configuration and extent of muscular control of the patient.

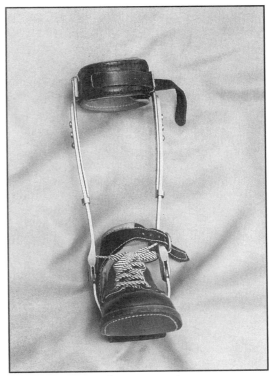

Figure 3-25a. Valgus correction strap—on a leather-metal AFO.

Mediolateral Control

To prevent the foot from supinating or pronating excessively, a varus- or valgus-correction strap can be added to a metal-leather AFO. The strap is T-shaped with the distal aspect of the strap attached to the shoe on one side and the proximal components buckling around the opposite upright (Figure 3-25a and 3-25b). A valgus-correction strap is sewn into the medial side of the shoe and buckled around the lateral upright. A varus-correction strap is sewn into the lateral side of the shoe and secured around the medial upright. Correction straps provide the same forces as the flanges in SA, but they add to donning time and may be secured too loosely or too tightly.

Uprights and Calf Bands

Most leather-metal AFOs have bilateral metal uprights that arise from the ankle joints and attach proximately to an upholstered metal or plastic calf band. Each upright should follow the contours of the patient's leg without touching the skin. A unilateral

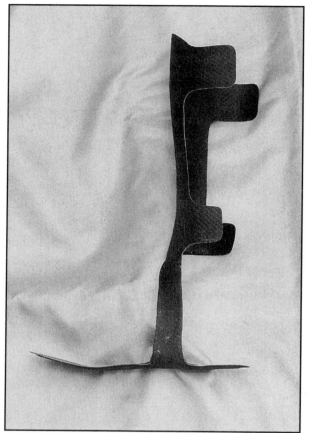

Figure 3-26. Camp ToeOFF Gait Rehabilitation Orthosis.

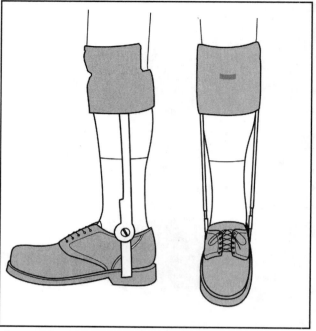

Figure 3-27a. Weight-relieving AFO—lateral and anterior views.

upright is less conspicuous but is subject to considerably more distal force than an upright that is half of a pair.

COMPOSITE MATERIALS

Composite materials made of graphite, various plastics, and titanium enable the design of orthoses that combine the best aspects of both plastic and leather-metal orthoses. The Camp ToeOFF Gait Rehabilitation Orthosis (Figure 3-26) is molded of carbon fiber, Kevlar (Pel Supply Company, Cleveland, Ohio), and fiberglass, making it thin, lightweight, and very durable. The orthosis has an anterior plate that covers the shin and a lateral strut from the distal end of the tibial plate to the middle of the lateral aspect of the foot plate. The orthosis functions like a rather flexible AFO-SA, permitting slight foot and ankle motion. Because the design provides flexible dorsiflexion resistance and ankle stabilization, indications for use include gastrocnemius weakness secondary to neuromuscular disorders

such as Charcot-Marie-Tooth disease, postpolio syndrome, and peripheral neuropathies. Contraindications include severe spasticity, severe edema, and diabetes with risk of ulceration from impaired protective sensation.

WEIGHT-RELIEVING ANKLE-FOOT ORTHOSES

A weight-relieving band on the AFO minimizes the forces going through the foot. In place of the calf shell or calf band, the weight-relieving AFO has a plastic circumferential brim molded to resemble a transtibial prosthetic socket, sometimes called patellar tendon bearing (PTB). The brim supports substantial load on the patellar ligament (Figures 3-27a and 3-27b). Load is transferred distally through the medial and lateral uprights, which terminate in a pair of limited motion ankle joints. The brim reduces but does not eliminate load through the tibia and foot. Complete unloading can only be achieved by keeping the foot off the floor as is accomplished in a KAFO with a patten bottom (see Chapter 4).

A weight-relieving AFO is occasionally used 2 to 6 weeks postfracture to replace a plaster cast (Figure 3-28). The orthosis has a tibial section made of a copolymer lined with closed-cell plastic foam that encases the leg from the knee to the ankle. Options for the shoe

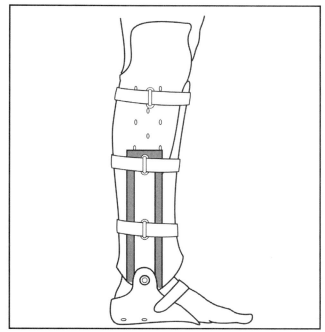

Figure 3-28. AFO designed to immobilize a tibial fracture.

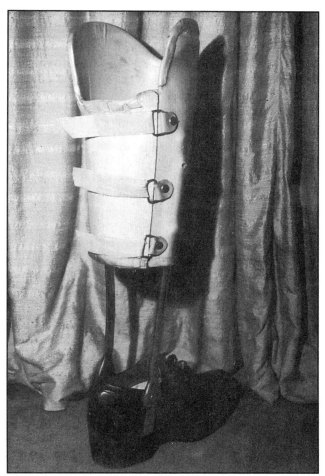

Figure 3-27b. Weight-relieving AFO—posterior aspect.

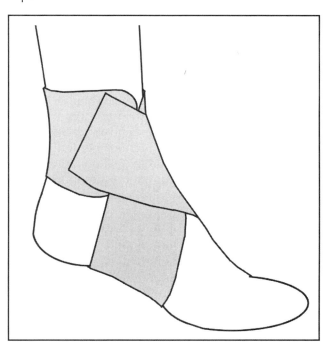

Figure 3-29. Elastic ankle support.

insert include a hinge or a solid ankle joint. The orthosis maintains compression for osseous alignment and edema control. Hook-and-pile closures facilitate fitting and can be adjusted for swelling.

FABRIC, LEATHER, AIR, AND GEL SUPPORTS

Many mass-produced orthoses provide stability at the ankle and foot. They are made of various fabrics and leather with pockets containing water, air, or gel. Fabric ankle supports can replace adhesive taping or elastic wrapping (Figure 3-29). Designs with lacing provide adaptability (Figure 3-30). Rigid vertical stays increase support. Air casts and splints are used to immobilize a limb that may be fractured, support an unstable or painful joint (Figure 3-31),[11] and reduce hypertonicity.[9,10] Some ankle supports have pockets containing gel (Figure 3-32) or ice (Figure 3-33) that can be cooled to control inflammation, edema, and pain.

CONTRACTURE-REDUCING AFOS

Some patients with Achilles' tendon contracture benefit from wearing an AFO that applies tensile stress to the posterior leg. Such orthoses have a coiled spring, elastic band, or an ankle joint with an

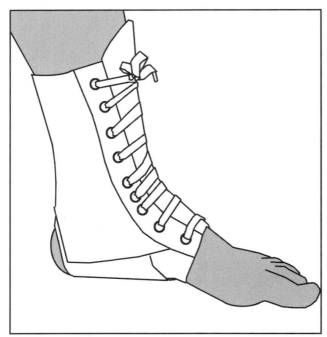

Figure 3-30. Canvas ankle support with lacing.

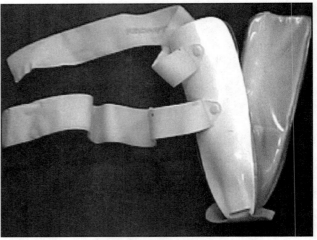

Figure 3-31. Air splint used to support a sprained or fractured ankle.

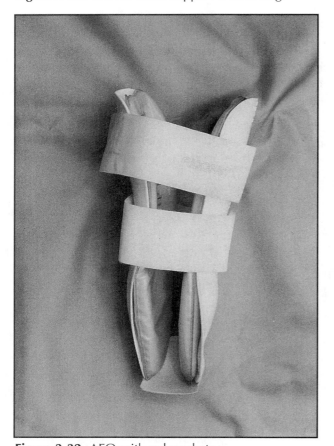

Figure 3-32. AFO with gel pockets.

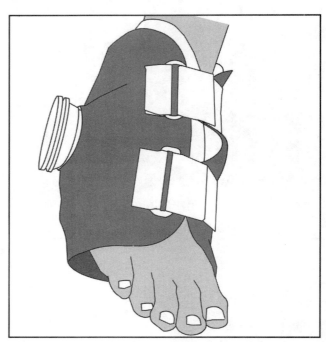

Figure 3-33. AFO with ice pockets.

adjustable mechanism.[12] As the contracture reduces, the clinician increases the tension on the ankle. Contracture-reducing AFOs are most effective when used in conjunction with an exercise program that emphasizes regaining mobility and strength in the antagonistic muscles.

GUIDELINES FOR PRESCRIPTION

The following are biomechanical guidelines to prescribing ankle-foot orthoses:
1. To provide plantar flexion control during swing phase
   a. AFO with dorsiflexion spring assist, either a PLS or a metal coil spring
   b. AFO with plantar flexion stop (plastic design)
   c. AFO-SA
   d. AFO with hinged ankle and a plantar flexion stop (leather metal design)
2. To provide dorsiflexion control during stance phase
   a. AFO-SA
   b. AFO with hinged ankle and a dorsiflexion stop (leather metal design)
   c. AFO with dorsiflexion stop (plastic design)
3. To provide foot mediolateral control during stance and swing phases
   a. AFO-SA
   b. AFO with solid ankle and medial (or lateral) flange
   c. Spiral or hemispiral AFO
   d. Valgus (or varus) control strap with AFO having a stirrup and lateral (or medial) uprights

SUMMARY

Plastic ankle-foot orthoses (AFOs) can be adapted to a variety of clinical needs, are relatively cosmetic and lightweight, and require little maintenance. They maintain close contact with the soft tissue contours of the leg but cannot be readily modified if leg contour changes. The most commonly prescribed AFOs include the PLS, which assists dorsiflexion; the SA, which restricts all foot and ankle motions; the hinged SA, which permits a variable amount of sagittal motion; and spiral and hemispiral orthoses, which provide moderate control of foot and ankle motion.

For patients with edema and dermatitis, leather-metal AFOs are more appropriate because they cover less skin and are somewhat more adjustable.

Composite designs, such as the Camp ToeOFF (Camp Healthcare, Atlanta, Ga), combine desirable features of plastic with the durability and strength of metal. For individuals who need less support, many mass-produced fabric orthoses are available. Some have water pockets or gel cells that can be cooled for control of soft tissue edema, inflammation, or pain. AFOs with adjustable ankle joints are indicated to reduce plantar flexion contracture.

THOUGHT QUESTIONS

1. Describe the forces in the three-point pressure system for the leather-metal AFO illustrated in Figure 3-16.
2. Describe the pressure system that controls supination in an AFO-SA with a lateral flange.
3. How can an AFO control genu recurvatum?
4. Why would you select a fabric ankle support rather than a plastic AFO for a patient with chronic ankle sprain?
5. How does the TIAFO interact with the foot and ankle throughout the gait cycle? Draw the ground reaction force acting during each portion of stance phase and the orthosis' reaction to these forces. Discuss the ankle motion and the congruency of the appliance with the skin throughout the gait cycle. Is the TIAFO effective for patients with moderate to severe spasticity? Explain your answer.

REFERENCES

1. Lin RS, Moore TJ. Orthoses for postpolio syndrome. In: Goldberg B, Hsu JD, eds. *Atlas of Orthoses and Assistive Devices*. 3rd ed. St. Louis, Mo: Mosby; 1997:455-458.
2. Lehman JF, Esselman PC, Ko MJ, Smith JC, de Lateur BJ, Dralle AJ. Plastic ankle-foot orthoses: evaluation of function. *Arch Phys Med Rehabil*. 1982;63:345-351.
3. Lehman JF, Condon SM, de Lateur BJ, Price R. Gait abnormalities in peroneal nerve paralysis and their corrections by orthoses: biomechanical study. *Arch Phys Med Rehabil*. 1986;67:380-386.
4. *Lower Limb Orthotics 1981 Revision*. New York, NY: New York University; 1986:129-136.
5. Perry J. *Gait Analysis: Normal and Pathological Function*. Thorofare, NJ: SLACK Incorporated; 1992:200-201.
6. Trautman P. Lower limb orthoses. In: Redford JB, Basmajian JV, Trautman P, eds. *In Orthotics: Clinical Practice and Rehabilitation Technology*. New York, NY: Churchill Livingstone; 1995:13-29.

7. Diamond MF, Ottenbacher KJ. Effect of a tone-inhibiting dynamic ankle-foot orthosis on stride characteristics of an adult with hemiparesis. *Phys Ther.* 1990;70:423-430.

8. Huber ST. Therapeutic application of orthotics. In: Umphred DA, ed. *Neurological Rehabilitation.* 2nd ed. St. Louis, Mo: CV Mosby; 1990:893-910.

9. Johnstone M. *Restoration of Normal Movement After Stroke.* Edinburgh: Churchill Livingstone; 1995:67,71-72,89.

10. Johnstone M. *Home Care for the Stroke Patient: Living in a Pattern.* 3rd ed. New York, NY: Churchill Livingstone; 1996:156-157,184.

11. Hals TMV, Sitler MR, Mattacola CG. Effect of a semi-rigid ankle stabilizer on performance in persons with functional ankle instability. *J Orthop Sports Phys Ther.* 2000;30:552-556.

12. Grissom SP, Blanton S. Treatment of upper motorneuron plantar flexion contractures by using an adjustable ankle-foot orthosis. *Arch Phys Med Rehabil.* 2001;82-270-273.

RECOMMENDED READING

1. Lehman JF, Condon SM, de Lateur BJ, Smith JC. Ankle-foot orthoses: effect on gait abnormalities in tibial nerve paralysis. *Arch Phys Med Rehabil.* 1985;66:212-218.

2. Lehman JF, Condon SM, de Lateur BJ, Smith JC. Gait abnormalities in tibial nerve paralysis: biomechanical study. *Arch Phys Med Rehabil.* 1985;66:80-85.

CASE STUDIES

For the following cases, select an appropriate orthosis, establish long- and short-term treatment goals, and develop a treatment plan.

- CF is an 18-year-old college student with a complete L4 spinal cord lesion, bilateral flaccid paralysis, and no joint contractures secondary to a motor vehicle accident. He would like to continue his studies in business administration.

- MO, an 83-year-old retired secretary, has unilateral tabes dorsalis with toe drag during swing phase and genu valgum. She has been using a leather-metal AFO with a dorsiflexion assist, a medial heel wedge, and varus correction strap for the past 20 years. The appliance is very worn, the dorsiflexion assist no longer functions, and the strap is torn. She would like a new AFO.

- SZ, a 77-year-old retired businessman, had a right cerebral vascular accident with left hemiplegia with severe extensor spasticity and clonus. He operated his own wholesale clothing business for 55 years, smoked two packs of cigarettes a day for 59 years, and has non-insulin dependent diabetes mellitus and hypertension. He lives with his wife in an apartment building that has an elevator.

- BN, a 2-year-old with spina bifida at the L5 level, has just started independent ambulation. She had two open-heart operations to correct a congenital heart defect. She has mild mental retardation.

- DS, a 65-year-old retired accountant, has left toe drag secondary to postpolio syndrome. He had poliomyelitis when he was 10 years old and was left with residual weakness in his left lower extremity. He had exercised daily but recently began getting weaker, so he stopped his program. He gained 50 pounds and now has difficulty walking around his house.

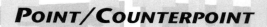

POINT/COUNTERPOINT

PA, a 44-year-old real estate agent, developed peroneal nerve palsy in her left lower extremity secondary to a diabetic neuropathy. She would like to continue working, but her disability has made it very difficult to show clients new properties.

JAN SAYS	JOAN SAYS

Orthotic Prescription

PA is concerned about her appearance and her gait. She will do well with a left AFO-PLS that will give her some dorsiflexion assistance. The orthosis allows some ankle motion, so she will have adequate plantar flexion during loading response and her shin can move over her fixed foot during midstance. The design will give her a little push-off assistance at the end of stance phase and will prevent toe drag during swing. Altogether, she will have a more efficient gait. To hold the brace on the leg and enable it to function, it must be worn in a low-heeled shoe that fastens high on the dorsum of the foot. The AFO-PLS has no moving parts and is made of durable plastic, so it requires very little maintenance.

PA is a busy, professional businesswoman who does a lot of walking. She needs an energy-efficient gait, and she needs to look good for her clients. I also recommend an AFO-PLS. It will give PA a gait pattern with minimal deviations. The orthosis is lightweight, easily hidden under pants or long skirts, and simple to put on and take off. She can slip it into any pair of low-heeled shoes that have a high closure on the dorsum, and she can change shoes daily to match her wardrobe.

Long-Term Goals

PA's program has three long-term goals:
- Safe, independent ambulation with the AFO-PLS on level surfaces, stairs, and ramps in the community.
- Independence in a diabetic foot care program to prevent lesions and possible amputation.
- Maintain full range of motion so that she will be able to achieve maximum benefit from the orthosis.

Every aspect of my physical therapy intervention will be done with consultation and consent from PA. I recommend two long-term goals for PA:
- Safe, independent ambulation with the AFO on level surfaces, stairs, and ramps in the community so that she can work with her clients and show them the properties.
- Independence in a diabetic foot care program to protect her feet from injury and prevent sequelae, such as ulcers, infections, and amputation.

Short-Term Goals

After 1 week of treatment, PA should be:
- Independent in donning and doffing the AFO-PLS
- Independent in ambulation with the AFO-PLS for 250 feet x 2
- Independent in self-stretching exercises to maintain foot and ankle ROM

My short-term goals for PA include:
- Ambulation with a mass-produced PLS with a straight cane and supervision; 100 feet x 2 in 1 week. This is to get her accustomed to wearing an orthosis and to build her walking endurance. As her gait improves and she gets more stable on her feet, she can stop using the cane.

JOAN SAYS   **JAN SAYS**

Short-Term Goals (Continued)

- Independence in donning and doffing the PLS in 1 week. She needs to be able to put on and take off the orthosis by herself. She also needs to know how to inspect her skin for abrasions, pressure areas, or skin lesions after wearing the orthosis. If she finds any abnormalities, she needs to know how to deal with them.
- Independence in a diabetic foot care program in 1 week. Proper foot hygiene is crucial for people with diabetes because they are at risk for developing gangrene and having amputations. I would teach PA how to test her sensation with a Siemmes-Weinstein monofilament, inspect her feet for lesions, select appropriate footwear, and maintain proper skin and nail care. Many diabetic amputations can be prevented with proper care. Two sensitive tests in identifying patients at risk for foot ulceration are clinical evaluations and the use of the Siemmes-Weinstein monofilament.
- Prescription for an AFO-PLS in 1 week. To achieve long-term goal, a prescription for the definitive orthosis.

Physical Therapy Plan

The treatment program will include the following:
- Donning and doffing instruction
- Patient education in diabetic foot care
- Gait training with the AFO-PLS
- Evaluation of her need for a cane
- Teaching self-range of motion exercises

To achieve the long- and short-term goals, the following treatment plan will be implemented:
- Gait training with PLS, straight cane, and supervision on level surfaces, ramps, and stairs within the confines of the therapy department; progressing to independent ambulation with PLS without a cane within the community; and finally progressing to independent ambulation with the AFO-PLS within the community
- Patient instruction in donning and doffing orthosis
- Patient education in diabetic foot care program
- Referral for an AFO-PLS prescription

Chapter 4

Knee-Ankle-Foot Orthoses and Knee Orthoses

"I have a pair of legs that only an orthopedic surgeon could love."
Joe Namath, *former star quarterback for the New York Jets*

With the development of new plastics, lighter and more durable metals, and better understanding of how limbs move through space, knee orthoses (KOs) have become more functional and more cosmetic. They serve a variety of clinical needs with a diversity of designs.

Two broad categories of KOs are those that are attached to AFOs, called knee-ankle-foot orthoses (KAFOs), and those that cross only the knee joint, called KOs. KAFOs enable substantial control of the lower limb. They are prescribed for patients with paralyzed muscles, fractures, or soft tissue laxity. KOs are indicated primarily for ligamentous laxity or for postoperative management to safeguard the joint during rehabilitation. Although athletes sometimes wear KOs to prevent or minimize injury during sports, this application remains controversial.

PLASTIC-METAL KAFOs

Most KAFOs have both plastic and metal components. Polypropylene is often used for the calf and thigh shells and the shoe insert. Metal, such as aluminum, magnesium, titanium, or steel, is used for the uprights. Joints are usually made of steel, which tolerates friction well. Plastic-metal orthoses with an insert foundation are easier to don than the older leather-metal designs, which included a stirrup riveted to the shoe.[1] Plastic-metal orthoses are substantially lighter in weight than metal-leather alternatives, resulting in faster walking at lower energy consumption.[2]

Shells

The distal aspect of the contemporary KAFO is usually a plastic AFO with a continuous calf shell with a shoe insert and a solid or hinged ankle. The most common proximal component is a plastic shell that covers the posterior thigh. The thigh shell is usually held on the limb with hook-and-pile straps. The shells create a streamlined, form-fitting contour that most patients prefer to older designs.[1] Occasionally, the KAFO includes a plastic bivalved circumferential component that encircles the thigh. The bivalved version reduces unit pressure on the anterior thigh but is more cumbersome to don and retains body heat. Regardless of the type of shell, the individual should wear a stocking or other fabric between the skin and the shell.

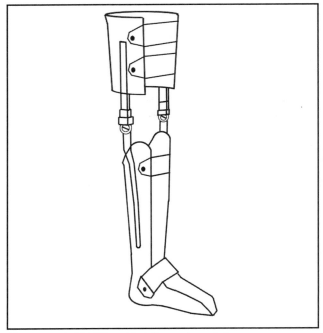

Figure 4-1. KAFO with bilateral uprights.

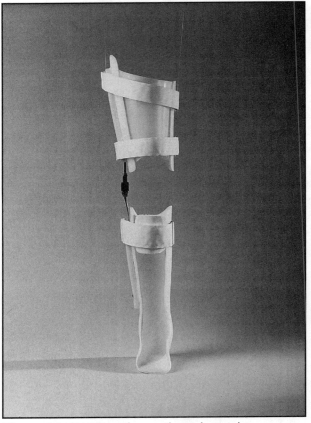

Figure 4-2. KAFO with a unilateral upright.

Uprights

Most KAFOs have bilateral metal uprights (Figure 4-1). For individuals who need control only in the frontal plane or who object to the conspicuousness of bilateral uprights, a unilateral upright (Figure 4-2) may suffice. The stress at the distal end of a unilateral upright, however, is considerable.

Knee Joints

Orthotic knee joints are either single-axis or polycentric. Single-axis joints offer a simple, inexpensive way of permitting motion at the knee when the wearer sits. They also permit motion at the knee during gait for some patients.

Active patients may find the single-axis knee joint inadequate because it allows pistoning, which can be irritative. The anatomical knee joint has a moving axis of rotation that cannot be tracked with a single-axis orthotic joint. Polycentric knee joints (Figure 4-3) offer a better approximation of natural knee motion, thereby avoiding pistoning and providing a better fit at all points in the knee flexion range. A secondary benefit of the polycentric knee joint is greater stability, so it does not always require a lock. The polycentric joint has more moving parts; requires more maintenance; and is heavier, bulkier, and more expensive than the single-axis joint.

The joint can be locked or unlocked. An unlocked joint provides mediolateral and rotational stability. It can be set straight within the uprights (Figure 4-4) or can be offset posteriorly to increase knee stability (Figure 4-5). For offset knee joints to be effective, the wearer must have no flexion contractures at the hip or knee and must walk on a level floor. A new unlocked knee joint features a microcomputer-controlled mechanism that stabilizes the knee during early stance.[3]

A dial knee joint (Figure 4-6) can be adjusted to permit motion within a predetermined arc.

Knee Locks

Most patients who need control in all planes require a knee joint with a lock. The most common design is a drop ring, which descends over a projection on the distal part of the joint to lock the joint in extension (Figure 4-7). Modifications of the drop lock include the addition of a spring-loaded retention button to prevent the ring from dropping inadvertently and a thigh-level spring-loaded release that the patient can use to raise the ring to flex the knee

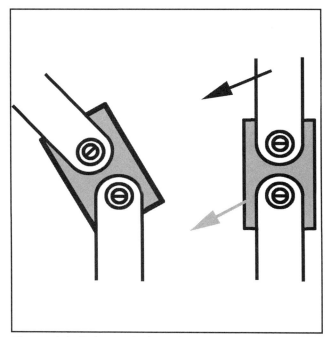

Figure 4-3. Polycentric knee joint.

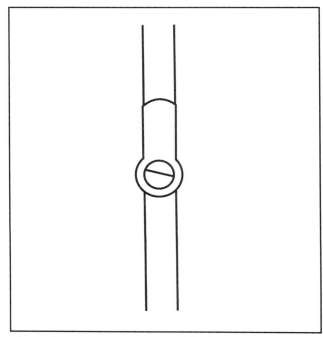

Figure 4-4. Knee joint set straight in uprights.

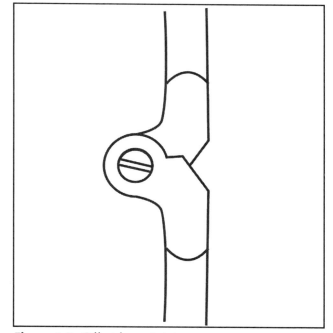

Figure 4-5. Offset knee joint.

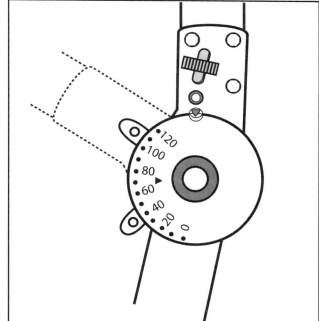

Figure 4-6. Dial knee joint.

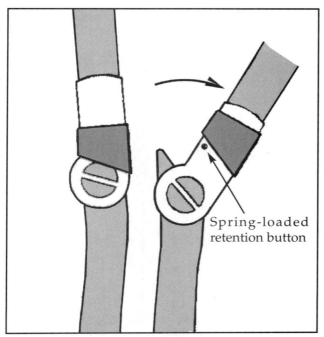

Figure 4-7. Drop ring lock.

Spring-loaded
retention button

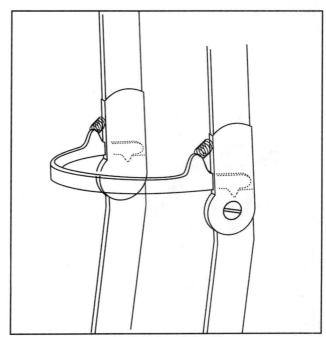

Figure 4-8. Pawl lock with a bail release.

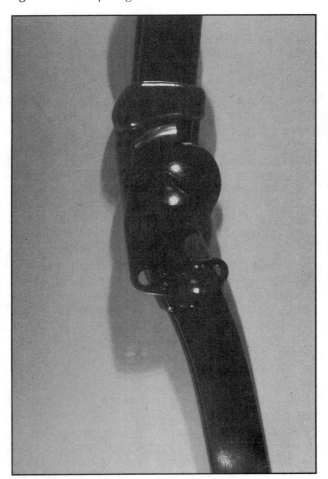

Figure 4-9. Fan lock.

during the sitting maneuver. Both uprights should be locked to maximize orthotic stability.

For individuals who cannot use a drop ring easily, perhaps because of hand weakness or poor balance, an alternative is a pawl lock with a bail release (Figure 4-8). When the patient presses the bail against a chair or other rigid surface or lifts the bail with one hand, the bail unlocks the medial and lateral knee joints so that the patient can flex the knee. The pawl lock with bail release provides simultaneous locking and unlocking of both uprights.

All of these locks require that the anatomical knee have full passive extension. A pawl lock or an ordinary drop ring lock cannot be engaged in the presence of knee flexion contracture. Special locks have been designed to stabilize the flexed knee. These locks provide for adjustment so that the clinician can match the angle of the orthotic knee joint to the angle of the anatomic knee. Occasionally, an adjustable lock is used therapeutically to reduce the contracture. The simplest adjustable lock is the fan lock (Figure 4-9), which provides five positions for angling the uprights; one inserts a screw in the appropriate hole to angle the uprights. The lock is secured with a drop ring. An alternative is the serrated lock (Figure 4-10), which includes a serrated disk on the distal upright and a drop ring lock. One can alter the alignment of the distal upright through a 360-degree range. Although more streamlined than the fan lock, the serrated lock may be contraindicat-

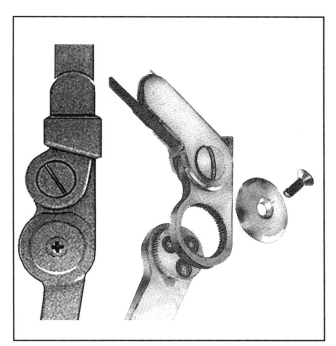

Figure 4-10. Serrated lock.

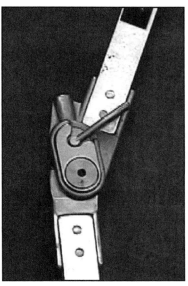

Figure 4-11. Ratchet lock (reproduced with permission of Orthotic Technical Supply).

ed in the presence of knee laxity. The lock displaces the angulation of the uprights several inches below the knee joint, imposing a posteriorly directed force on the anatomic knee. A ratchet lock, such as the Step Lock (Figure 4-11), is another option. The locking projection lodges in a depression in the ratchet to secure the joint. This component is bulkier and more expensive than fan or serrated locks.

Knee Bands and Pads

In addition to some type of knee lock, the patient with knee extensor paralysis requires an anterior component in the vicinity of the knee. The component may be a rigid suprapatellar (Figure 4-12) or a pretibial band (Figure 4-13), both of which impose a posteriorly directed force to stabilize the knee. They do not interfere with sitting and are relatively easy to don. A leather kneepad (Figure 4-14) usually has four straps buckled to the medial and lateral uprights above and below the knee joint. Strap tension is adjustable, but the component impedes knee flexion when the wearer tries to sit, is cumbersome, and takes a longer time to don.

Frontal Plane Control

Most KAFOs are prescribed for patients with knee extensor paralysis who need sagittal plane control. Orthoses are sometimes beneficial for individuals with soft tissue laxity, such as occurs in severe arthritis. These devices control the knee in the frontal plane and occasionally in the transverse plane as well. For the adult with genu valgum, for example, the KAFO may have an extension of the plastic calf

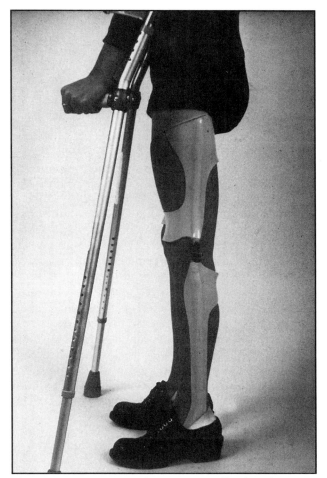

Figure 4-12. KAFO with a suprapatellar band.

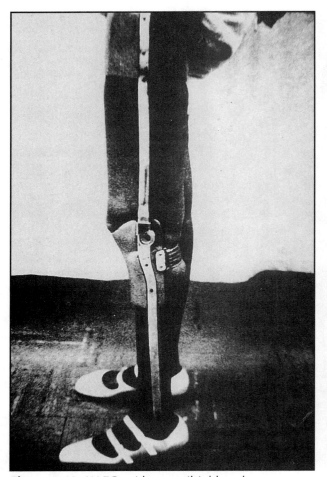

Figure 4-13. KAFO with a pretibial band.

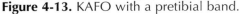

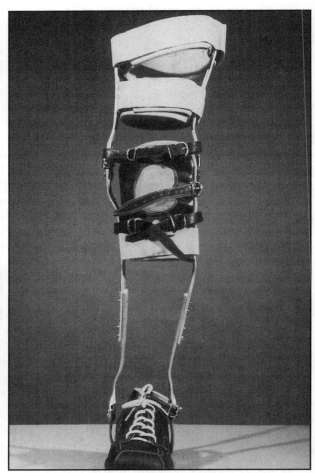

Figure 4-14. KAFO with leather knee pad.

shell on the medial side. A mild frontal plane defor-mity can be controlled with an AFO with an extend-ed calf shell. Alternative methods are less satisfacto-ry. For genu valgum, for example, the leather knee pad, having a medial extension with a buckled strap, is buckled around the lateral upright to provide a lat-erally directed force. The additional strap increases donning time, and the posterior portion of the strap tends to lodge uncomfortably in the popliteal fossa when the wearer sits. The same deformity has been addressed with an upholstered disk attached to the medial upright near the knee joint. The disk also applies a laterally directed force. Although the disk does not interfere with donning or with sitting com-fort, it imposes high pressure on the medial side of the knee when the wearer stands.

A mechanical knee joint, whether single-axis or polycentric, on either a KAFO or KO interferes with anatomic motion. During walking, the anatomic knee moves in all three planes[4,5] with a subtlety that no current mechanical knee joint can match.[6] If the orthotic joint is unlocked, some pistoning with shear-ing force is inevitable. If the joint is locked, the wear-er has a conspicuously altered gait, encounters diffi-culty when rising from a chair and sitting, sustains increased ground reaction forces,[7] and incurs increased oxygen cost when walking.[8,9] Assuming a unilateral orthosis, the increased metabolic demand and resulting gait deviation can be minimized by a 1 cm lift placed on the contralateral shoe sole[10] or by applying the stabilizing force as close to the center of the knee as possible.[11] Because of the drawbacks of both locked and unlocked knee joints, an AFO should be used instead of a KAFO whenever possible.[12,13]

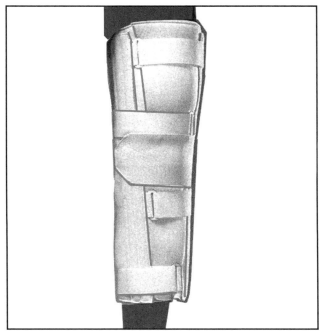

Figure 4-15. KO immobilizer with no knee joint.

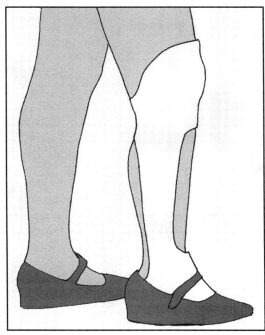

Figure 4-16. Supracondylar KAFO.

KNEE IMMOBILIZERS

The KAFO or KO can be designed without a mechanical knee joint to hold the knee in full extension (Figure 4-15). Immobilizer splints are usually made of canvas with vertical metal stays for additional rigidity. Those that cover most of the thigh and leg are used for immediate management of trauma and hemophiliac hemorrhage.

SUPRACONDYLAR KAFOs

The supracondylar KAFO (Figure 4-16) stabilizes the knee, ankle, and foot. The proximal portion encases the knee to provide support in all three planes. The anterior proximal shell and the foot segment impose posteriorly directed forces that counteract the anteriorly directed force exerted by the calf band. The three-point pressure system resists genu recurvatum during stance phase while permitting knee flexion during swing phase and during sitting. The distal portion of the orthosis immobilizes the ankle, hindfoot, and midfoot in slight plantar flexion, so a knee extension moment is generated during the stance phase of gait. By encircling the foot and ankle, the orthosis prevents foot motion, which further stabilizes the knee. Consequently, no mechanical knee lock is needed. The orthosis has durable construction without any moving parts. The streamlined design is aesthetically pleasing, although the edge of the proximal shell protrudes above the thigh when the patient sits, so the orthosis cannot be worn under tight trousers or a snugly fitting skirt. The shoe should have a rocker bar to maintain forward momentum during walking. A mechanical knee joint can be added to allow knee flexion to improve sitting appearance, but the joint adds bulk, weight, cost, and fragility. The supracondylar KAFO is contraindicated in the presence of fluctuating edema because the patient cannot adjust the snugness of the orthosis.

WEIGHT-RELIEVING ORTHOSES

A thigh shell extended to the ischium provides the maximum support available from a KAFO. Such shells are usually quadrilateral in shape to control rotation. An ischial seat or ring is incorporated in the design to transfer force from the pelvis onto the uprights of the brace for partial unloading of the leg. If complete unloading is required, the KAFO must include an ischial seat and a patten bottom, which is a hoof-like projection attached to the distal uprights (Figure 4-17). The patten bottom raises the shoe off the floor, preventing the patient from weightbearing through the foot. The contralateral shoe requires a lift to maintain a level pelvis.

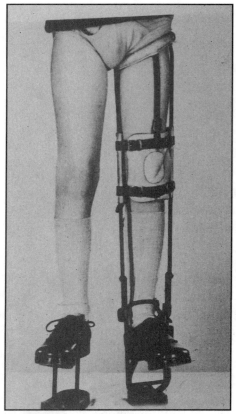

Figure 4-17. Weight-relieving KAFO.

FRACTURE ORTHOSES

An alternative to immobilizing a fractured limb in plaster or fiberglass is a fracture orthosis (Figure 4-18). It is indicated especially for distal femoral or tibial plateau fractures that are treated either operatively or nonoperatively. The mass-produced orthoses have polyethylene thigh and calf shells with hook-and-pile fasteners. The shells compress the limb to maintain bony alignment and minimize edema. Unlike casts, fracture orthoses enable inspection of the limb. They can be fitted with a variety of orthotic knee joints depending on the extent of knee excursion desired. The foot and ankle component can be a solid ankle shoe insert to prevent ankle and foot motion or an insert that allows dorsiflexion and plantar flexion while restraining midfoot motion.

LEATHER-METAL KAFOS

Although plastic-metal KAFOs and KOs are more common, both leather-metal and plastic designs

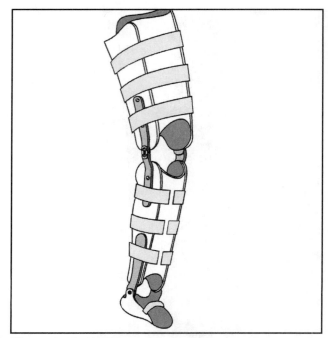

Figure 4-18. KAFO used in fracture management.

enable comparable function.[1] Leather-metal orthoses (Figure 4-19) are required for the individual who has severe edema and fluctuating leg volume. They are more readily adjustable by the patient.

Leather-metal KAFOs usually have aluminum calf and thigh bands upholstered with felt and covered with horsehide. Because metal is stronger and more rigid than plastic, the metal bands can be narrower than the plastic ones. Consequently, less skin surface is covered. Some people find this more comfortable than being encased in plastic, especially in warm weather. The same joints that are used in plastic-metal KAFOs can be installed in the leather-metal designs.[14]

KNEE ORTHOSES

KO designs have four main applications: functional, rehabilitative, prophylactic, and contracture-reducing.[15] A functional KO supports the anatomic knee that has soft tissue laxity or weakened or paralyzed muscles. Rehabilitative orthoses are prescribed as part of an active treatment program, such as after surgical repair of a ligament. Prophylactic KOs are intended to prevent knee injuries, primarily in vigorous sports. Other KOs are supportive, designed to assist in patellar tracking, and relieve patellar chondromalacia.

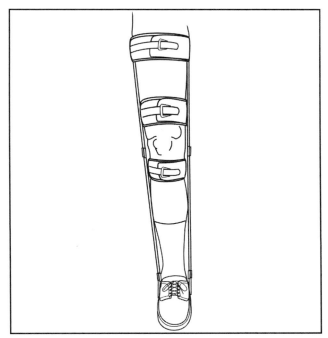

Figure 4-19. Leather-metal KAFO.

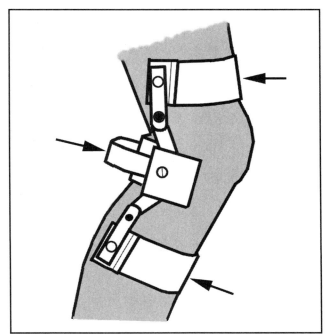

Figure 4-20. Swedish knee cage KO providing antero-posterior support.

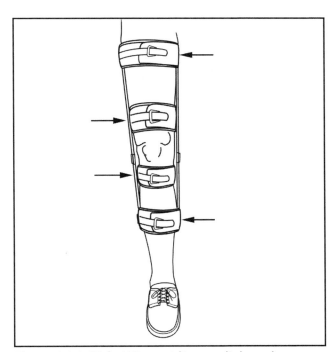

Figure 4-21. Right KO providing mediolateral support.

Functional KOs

For the person with an unstable knee, a KO may increase stability enough to enable ordinary function.[16] Most KOs have bilateral uprights made of metal, fiberglass, or plastic. Shells encasing the thigh and leg are made of plastic laminate or composites, metal, leather, or fabric.

Functional KOs can have polycentric or single-axis knee joints and can come with or without locks. KOs have been designed to provide anteroposterior support for ligamentous instability (Figure 4-20), mediolateral support for genu varum and valgum (Figure 4-21), and rotational support (Figure 4-22). Manufacturers of some functional KOs let wearers choose the color and pattern of the shells so that they can match their exercise outfits.

The Swedish knee cage (see Figure 4-20) helps to stabilize the knee when an individual is first learning to walk after a stroke. It has no moving parts, so it is durable and easy to use. It has metal uprights, anterior thigh and shin bands, and a posterior pad for the popliteal region. The thigh and shin bands are made of webbing or heavy elastic. During stance phase, this KO prevents the knee from hyperextending. As the patient walks faster, the lack of a mechanical knee joint causes the KO to slip or rotate and its stabilizing function decreases. Like the supracondylar AFO, the proximal edge of the Swedish knee cage protrudes when the wearer is seated.

Rehabilitative KOs

Knee orthoses are often used following knee surgery. These orthoses are designed for short-term use

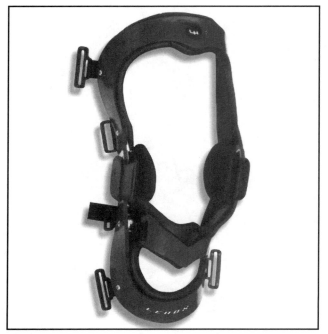

Figure 4-22. KO providing rotational support.

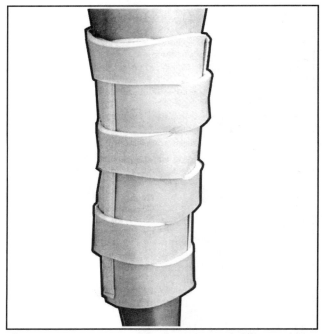

Figure 4-23. Postoperative knee immobilizer with no mechanical joint.

while the patient is undergoing rehabilitation and are discontinued when treatment is completed. The simplest designs are constructed of canvas with or without foam backing. Short, unjointed immobilizers (Figure 4-23) have metal stays to hold the knee in extension. Hook-and-pile straps with or without D-rings secure the orthosis in place. More sophisticated appliances have leg and thigh bands constructed of webbing, semirigid nylon, or a composite fiber, and may have a dial lock to let the clinician set the permitted range of motion. Rehabilitative KOs may have single or polycentric knee joints that may or may not lock.

Prophylactic KOs

The most controversial KOs are those prescribed to prevent injury. The literature offers conflicting studies about their effectiveness. Sitler et al[17] found that prophylactic KOs did reduce the total number of knee injuries in football players, but the benefits were dependent on the players' positions. Defensive players who wore KOs had fewer injuries, but offensive players did not. Albright et al[18] conducted an extensive literature review and concluded that athletes wearing prophylactic KOs were less likely to incur sprains of the anterior cruciate ligament. Some researchers reported that prophylactic knee bracing

had no effect on reducing injuries,[19] while others found that the KOs increased the number of injuries,[20] probably by altering neuromuscular control.[21]

Contracture-Reducing KOs

For individuals with knee contractures, a variety of KOs can help restore range of motion. Most have bilateral uprights and apply a constant force to the knee. For nonambulatory patients, an adjustable hinged knee joint allows incremental increases in joint range of motion (Figure 4-24). Some KOs have knee joints with springs, which exert more tensile force on the anatomic knee as compared with knee units that lack springs. More force can be applied and easier adjustments made with a turnbuckle mechanism (Figure 4-25), as greater range is achieved. KOs for contracture management have thigh and calf bands made of fabric, metal, or plastic. One design has two air bladders behind the knee that can be inflated to maximize pressure distribution. These designs can be used to reduce either flexion or extension contractures. Other joints have an elastic component in the form of a coiled spring or elastic band that provides tensile stress across the joint.

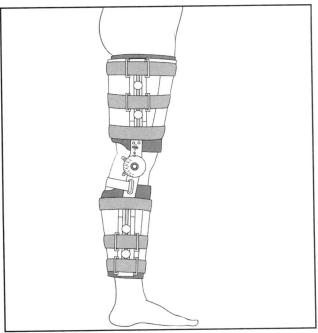

Figure 4-24. KO with adjustable hinges.

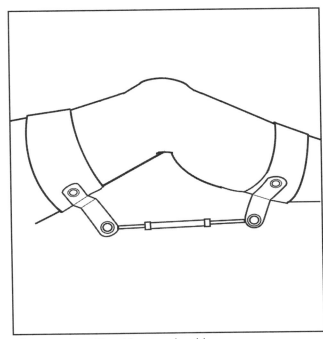

Figure 4-25. KO with a turnbuckle.

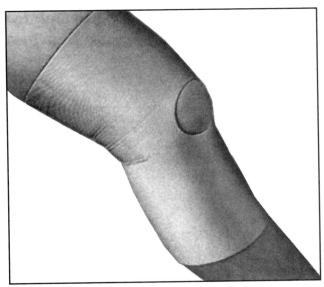

Figure 4-26. Neoprene sleeve.

Supportive KOs

To provide moderate support to the joint, assist in patellar tracking, and relieve patellar chondromalacia, several fabric KOs are available. They are made of cotton or synthetic canvas with or without elastic panels, rigid reinforcements, or neoprene. Some patients develop an allergic contact dermatitis to neoprene.[22] The simplest design is an elastic sleeve that surrounds the knee (Figure 4-26). The sleeve can be modified with pads, uprights, and hook-and-pile

straps to provide the desired support. The sleeve improves the accuracy of knee flexion.[23] Other modifications include an opening for the patella or the addition of a gel pad that can be heated or cooled to provide a thermal effect.

Johnstone[24,25] recommended the use of a double-chamber air splint and a "leg gaiter" (Figure 4-27) for patients with hemiplegia to encourage weight-bearing through the involved leg with a slightly flexed knee. The splint stabilizes the knee, inhibits spasticity, and controls extensor thrust. Although she noted that "the gaiter is not intended as a splint for walking,"[24] she presented a case study in which a patient used the gaiter for gait training on level surfaces and stairs.[25]

GUIDELINES FOR PRESCRIPTION

The following are biomechanical guidelines for prescribing foot, ankle-foot, knee-ankle-foot, and knee orthoses.
1. To control quad weakness during the stance phase
   a. Low shoe heel
   b. AFO-SA set in plantar flexion
   c. AFO-SA and anterior proximal band
   d. KAFO with a knee lock and prepatellar or suprapatellar band or knee pad
   e. KAFO with a dial joint

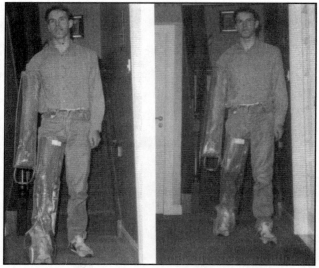

Figure 4-27. KO with air-filled chambers; air sleeve; AFO with air chambers (reprinted from Johnstone M. *Home Care for the Stroke Patient: Living in a Pattern.* 3rd ed. New York, NY: Churchill Livingstone; 1996 by permission of the publisher Churchill Livingstone).

2. To control knee flexion during the stance phase in the presence of knee flexion contracture
   a. KAFO with a fan knee lock
   b. KAFO with a ratchet lock (eg, Step Lock)
   c. KAFO with a serrated knee lock
3. To control knee hyperextension during the stance phase in the presence of genu recurvatum
   a. Slightly higher shoe heel
   b. AFO-SA set in dorsiflexion
   c. KAFO with a posteriorly offset calf and distal thigh bands
   d. Swedish knee cage
4. To provide mediolateral control during the stance phase in the presence of genu valgum
   a. AFO-SA with a rigid extended calf band on the medial side
   b. KAFO with a rigid extended calf band on the medial side; orthosis may or may not have a knee lock
   c. KAFO with a knee lock and knee pad with the fifth strap buckled on the lateral upright
   d. KAFO with a medial disk at the knee

SUMMARY

KAFOs and KOs serve to stabilize and occasionally to immobilize the leg. Plastic-metal designs combine the light, cosmetic qualities of plastic for the shells with the durability of metal for the uprights and mechanical joints. Plastic-metal KAFOs meet the needs of most patients who have knee impairments but cannot accommodate limbs that have severe edema with changing volume. Leather-metal KAFOs are less form-fitting, so they tolerate more limb volume change. Joints may be single-axis or polycentric and may be secured with a drop ring lock or other system that limits joint range of motion. KO designs can be classified as functional, rehabilitative, prophylactic, or contracture-reducing. Functional KOs compensate for soft tissue laxity or muscles that are weakened or paralyzed. Rehabilitative KOs are prescribed as part of a rehabilitation program, following surgery. Prophylactic KOs are intended to prevent athletic knee injuries.

THOUGHT QUESTIONS

1. Design a plastic KAFO for a patient with severe osteoarthritis, an unstable knee, and genu valgum. Include a description of all components.
2. Design a plastic KO for a patient with severe osteoarthritis, an unstable knee, and genu valgum. Include a description of all components. Compare your design with that in the previous question. What major factors would you consider when deciding to prescribe a KAFO rather than a KO for this patient?
3. Rigid designs, made either of polypropylene or metal, were once popular for controlling genu recurvatum. The Swedish knee cage and a plastic supracondylar KAFO proved to be less effective than other designs in countering hyperextension. List three reasons why and explain each.
4. Some clinicians believe that a KAFO is excessive bracing and argue that most knee disorders can be managed either with an AFO or a KO. Take a position on this issue and defend it.
5. You are a physical therapist working with a women's high school field hockey team. The coach tells you that the players had quite a few knee injuries last season and that she would like to prevent as many injuries as possible this year. She shows you a picture of a KO and tells you that she read an article in a sports journal explaining that this brace can prevent knee injuries. Each orthosis costs $800. While it would be very expensive to buy a pair of KOs for each member of the team, she thinks buying

one pair would be worthwhile if she can prevent her star player from getting injured. She wants to know your opinion. What will you tell her?

REFERENCES

1. Krebs DE, Edelstein JE, Fishman S. Comparison of plastic/metal and leather/metal knee-ankle-foot orthoses. *Am J Phys Med Rehabil.* 1988;67:175-185.

2. Taktak DM, Bowker P. Lightweight, modular knee-ankle-foot orthosis for Duchenne's muscular dystrophy: design, development, and evaluation. *Arch Phys Med Rehabil.* 1995;76:1156-1162.

3. Suga T, Kameyama O, Ogawa R, Matsuura M, Oka H. Newly designed computer controlled knee-ankle-foot orthosis (Intelligent Orthosis). *Prosthet Orthot Int.* 1998;22:230-239.

4. Kettelcamp DB, Johnson RJ, Smidt GL, Chao EY, Walker M. An electrogoniometric study of knee motion in normal gait. *J Bone Joint Surg [Am].* 1970;52:775-790.

5. Levens AS, Inman VT, Blosser JA. Transverse rotation of the segments of the lower extremity in locomotion. *J Bone Joint Surg [Am].* 1948;30:859-872.

6. Bahler A. Fundamental biomechanical principles in the orthotic treatment of the knee. *Journal of Prosthetics and Orthotics.* 1992;4:157-165.

7. Cook TM, Farrell KP, Carey IA, Gibbs JM, Wiger GE. Effects of restricted knee flexion and walking speed on the vertical ground reaction force during gait. *J Orthop Sports Phys Ther.* 1997;25:236-244.

8. Abdulhadi HM, Kerrigan DC, LaRaia PJ. Contralateral shoe-lift: effect on oxygen cost of walking with an immobilized knee. *Arch Phys Med Rehabil.* 1996;77:670-672.

9. Perry J. *Gait Analysis: Normal and Pathological Function.* Thorofare, NJ: SLACK Incorporated; 1992:467-469.

10. Kerrigan DC, Abdulhadi HM, Ribaudo TA, Della Crose U. Biomechanical effects of a contralateral shoe-lift on walking with an immobilized knee. *Arch Phys Med Rehabil.* 1997;78:1085-1091.

11. Lehmann JF, Warren CG. Restraining forces in various designs of knee-ankle orthoses: their placement and effect on the anatomical knee joint. *Arch Phys Med Rehabil.* 1976;57:430-437.

12. Huber ST. Therapeutic application of orthotics. In: Umphred DA, ed. *Neurological Rehabilitation.* 2nd ed. St. Louis, Mo: CV Mosby; 1990:893-910.

13. Nielsen J. Limiting KAFO use to maximize free movement. *Biomechanics.* 1995;2:31-35.

14. *Lower Limb Orthotics.* New York, NY: New York University; 1986:137-142, 148-156.

15. American Academy of Orthopaedic Surgeons. Knee braces. In: Derz DJ, ed. *Seminar Report.* Chicago, Ill: American Academy of Orthopaedic Surgeons; 1985.

16. Schlegel TF, Steadman JR. Knee orthoses for sports-related disorders. In: Goldberg B, Hsu JD, eds. *Atlas of Orthoses and Assistive Devices.* 2nd ed. St. Louis, Mo: Mosby; 1997:415-426.

17. Sitler M, Ryan J, Hopkinson J, Kolb R, Polley D. The efficacy of a prophylactic knee brace to reduce knee injuries in football: a prospective, randomized study at West Point. *Am J Sports Med.* 1990;18:310-315.

18. Albright JP, Saterbak A, Stokes A. Use of knee braces in sports: current recommendations. *Sports Med.* 1995;20:281-301.

19. Wu GKH, Ng GYF, Mak AFT. Effects of knee bracing on the functional performance of patients with anterior cruciate ligament reconstruction. *Arch Phys Med Rehabil.* 2001;82:282-285.

20. Teitz C, Hermanson B, Kronmal R, Diehr P. Evaluation of the use of braces to prevent injury to the knee in collegiate football players. *J Bone Joint Surg [Am].* 1987;69:2-9.

21. Ostering LR, Robertson RN. Effects of prophylactic knee bracing on lower extremity joint position and muscle activation during running. *Am J Sports Med.* 1993;21:733-737.

22. Lazarov A, Ingber A. Textile dermatitis from Disperse Blue 85 in a knee brace. *Contact Dermatitis.* 1998;38:357.

23. McNair PJ, Stanley SN, Strauss GR. Knee bracing: effects on proprioception. *Arch Phys Med Rehabil.* 1996;77:287-289.

24. Johnstone M. *Restoration of Normal Movement after Stroke.* Edinburgh: Churchill Livingstone; 1995:68-69.

25. Johnstone M. *Home Care for the Stroke Patient: Living in a Pattern.* 3rd ed. New York, NY: Churchill Livingstone; 1996:182-183, 207, 211.

26. Glancy J. *Orthotic Recommendations: Management of Functional Forefoot Drop.* Indianapolis, Ind: Department of Publishing, Document and Distribution Services at Indiana University-Purdue University; 2000.

RECOMMENDED READING

Trautman P. Lower limb orthoses. In: Redford JB, Basmajian JV, Trautman P, eds. *Orthotics: Clinical Practice and Rehabilitation Technology.* New York, NY: Churchill Livingstone; 1995:13-29.

For the following cases, select an appropriate orthosis, establish long- and short-term treatment goals, and develop a treatment plan.

- MK, a 16-year-old gymnast, tore her medial meniscus while dismounting from the uneven bars. She had arthroscopic surgery to remove the torn meniscus, and the surgeon prescribed a KO to protect the knee during her rehabilitation. The surgeon does not want her knee to move more than 90 degrees from full extension to 90 degrees flexion.

- HR, a 67-year-old dentist, had a left total knee replacement (TKR) secondary to severe osteoarthritis. He had a TKR on his right knee last year and now has 0 to 90 degrees of active range of motion in his right knee. All muscles around the right knee are in the good (4/5) range. Immediately after the left TKR, he had trace (1/5) muscle strength in his left quadriceps and hamstring muscles. He has active range of motion at the left knee between 25 and 55 degrees of flexion. Swelling and pain limit range.

- FC, a 64-year-old homemaker, had poliomyelitis when she was 6 years old. The disease weakened all of the muscles in her left lower extremity, and the limb is 4 cm shorter than the right lower extremity. Her left knee has severe ligamentous laxity and exhibits 25 degrees of recurvatum on weight-bearing. All muscle groups in the left foot and ankle are in the trace (1/5) range. The left quadriceps and hamstring muscles are poor (2/5). The left ankle lacks 5 degrees of passive dorsiflexion. The right lower extremity has active range of motion within normal limits and muscle strengths within the normal (5/5) range. She has used a leather-metal KAFO with bilateral Lofstrand crutches since she was a child. She says that she is a household ambulator. Her KAFO is now very worn. The leather strap stabilizing the calf band and the leather pad supporting the knee have torn. The single-axis knee joint with a drop ring has a broken spring retention release. She has a leather shoe with laces, a Blucher-style opening, and a heel lift to accommodate the plantar flexion contracture and leg-length discrepancy. The shoe is attached to the KAFO by a solid stirrup. The leather over the toe box has cracked and the sole under the metatarsal heads has a hole. She is comfortable with her current KAFO, although it needs to be repaired. She would consider a new orthosis if it would work better than her current one.

- QH, a 76-year-old volunteer in a senior center, has severe osteoarthritis of her right knee. She has bilateral genu valgum with considerable instability of the medial collateral and anterior cruciate ligaments. She walks with a slow, antalgic gait and wants to be more active, since she is now gaining weight.

- NJ, a 79-year-old who had a right cerebral vascular accident 8 months ago and now has left hemiplegia, has been referred to your clinic for rehabilitation. Her left lower extremity has a moderate extensor thrust, and she demonstrates excessive plantar flexion and inversion, genu recurvatum, inadequate knee flexion during stance, and a flexion withdrawal pattern during swing. Her left hip abductors are weak, and she walks with her left pelvis retracted.

POINT/COUNTERPOINT

PL, a 47-year-old film editor, has pain on the medial aspect of both patellae. She has bilateral positive drawer signs and laxity of both medial collateral and anterior cruciate ligaments. Passive range of motion is within normal limits, and all knee muscles bilaterally are in the normal (5/5) range. Crepitus is present in both knees, and both patellae deviate laterally during knee extension. She exhibits bilateral midfoot hyperpronation from loading response through terminal stance. PL would like some relief from the knee pain.

JOAN SAYS	JAN SAYS

Orthotic Prescription

I recommend bilateral UCBLs to control the hyperpronation. To wear these orthoses, PL needs extra-depth shoes with snug-fitting counters. To absorb shock, the shoes should have resilient heels and soles.

The problem at her knees stems from the hyperpronation at her feet. I would use bilateral UCBLs to control midfoot hyperpronation and genu valgus. To assist with shock-absorption, I recommend lateral cushion heel wedges built into the soles of both shoes.[26]

Long-Term Goals

The long-term goal for PL is pain-free gait.

I always set goals with my patients, so, with the collaboration of PL, I would like to see PL have the following at the end of physical therapy intervention:
- Pain-free gait
- Control of midfoot hyperpronation bilaterally

Short-Term Goals

I want to make PL more comfortable right away, take some of the stress off her knees, and get a prescription for her orthoses. Goals for the first week of therapy include:
- Reduce knee pain from 9/10 to 5/10
- Stabilize feet to decrease force on the knees
- Prescription for well-fitting shoes and UCBLs

To achieve the long-term goals, I would set the following three short-term goals to be accomplished during the first week of intervention:
- Reduce knee pain from 9/10 to 5/10
- Stabilize knees and feet
- Prescribe UCBLs with lateral cushion heel wedges in both shoes

JOAN SAYS	JAN SAYS

Treatment Plan

PL's treatment plan must minimize her pain and stabilize her knees. The program should include the following:

- Bilateral quadriceps strengthening exercises to improve her stability
- Heat, elevation, and compression to decrease knee pain and inflammation
- Referral for UCBLs and shoes to stabilize her legs
- Modify PL's recreational activities to allow pain to resolve

To achieve the long-term goals, I recommend the following intervention:

- Taping both knees with athletic tape to control patellar tracking and both longitudinal arches to control hyperpronation. Initially, I would do the taping and then I would teach the technique to PL
- Bilateral quadriceps strengthening exercises to help stabilize the knees
- Heat or other modality for knee pain
- Referral for prescription for bilateral UCBLs with lateral heel wedges on the shoes' soles

Chapter 5

Orthoses for Paraplegia and Hip Disorders

"...before he gave up the idea of standing during his speeches, I went into his bedroom and found him with his braces on, walking up and down, leaning on the arm of Dr. McIntire. He was literally trying to learn to walk again!... In spite of the almost overwhelming amount of work that faced him daily in late 1944, he had made up his mind that he was going to walk again—and he did. I never saw such a display of guts."

Judge Samuel Rosenman, *In FDR's Splendid Deception, Hugh Gregory Gallagher*

Restoration of walking is the goal sought by both patients who have paraplegia and by clinicians. Various orthoses and other interventions have been designed to achieve this objective. The biomechanical problem involved with walking has two somewhat contradictory elements, namely providing static upright balance and dynamic balance as the patient voluntarily controls motion. The issue is further complicated by physiological concerns, principally the level and completeness of the spinal cord lesion and such factors as the presence of contractures, obesity, severe spasticity, sensory loss, and depression.

Patients who have hip disorders pose a different problem. Some may be treated with orthoses. Candidates for hip orthoses (HOs) are usually older adults who are recovering from hip surgery or who require some means of limiting hip motion to a pain-free range. Occasionally, hip orthoses are prescribed for children who lack hip control.

PARAPLEGIA

The individual with spinal cord disorder, typically a child with spina bifida or a man with a spinal cord injury, who wishes to walk must have a means of achieving a secure standing position and a way of moving from place to place in an energy-efficient manner.

Orthoses designed for standing apply a four-point force system to the wearer, namely posteriorly directed forces at the midchest and midleg and anteriorly directed forces from the dorsolumbar region and feet (Figure 5-1). The patient must have sufficient control of the upper torso, neck, and head in order to stand. Control can be achieved by voluntary muscular control, operative fixation of the cervical and upper thoracic spine, or a cervical orthosis. The standing orthosis must also provide a stable base. The base may be an orthotic foundation, either a pair of plastic shoe inserts or steel stirrups each with an ankle control that restricts mediolateral and posterior motion, and may also limit anterior motion. An alternative base is a flat foundation to which shoes are secured. Stability is enhanced by the use of a walker, crutches, parallel bars, or a harness attached to an overhead rigid frame. Some patients prefer to lean against a sink or other immovable object. Alternatives to a standing orthosis include a wheelchair with a mechanism that enables the occupant to rise and electrical stimulation of the hip and knee extensors.[1]

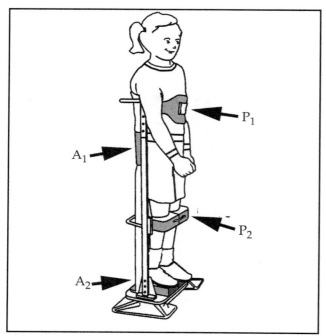

Figure 5-1. Four-point force system needed for orthotically assisted standing.

Standing has many benefits, for it stresses the skeleton, reducing the risk of disuse osteoporosis. Upright posture also fosters digestion, respiration, urinary drainage, and is associated with fewer fractures and decubitus ulcers. Psychologically, the patient is now at eye level with peers. The work area increases if the person has sufficient balance to be able to reach into overhead cabinets and shelves.

The individual who has a lesion in the thoracic or lumbar level of the spinal cord will have great difficulty achieving functional locomotion (ie, being able to move easily and independently in the community). Lacking voluntary control of the hips, knees, and ankles, the patient must use muscles of the upper trunk and neck together with the upper limbs to shift weight from the swinging leg and then advance it. Very seldom can the person expect to walk outdoors or maneuver over stairs, ramps, and other common environmental features, regardless of orthosis type. Orthotically assisted gait, however, enables some people to move about indoors, particularly in locations in which a wheelchair is too bulky. The gait is slower than that of nondisabled persons and the energy cost is higher. Nevertheless, patients report enjoying the ability to resume some mode of walking, looking face-to-face with other people, and being able to evaluate directly whether the effort needed to ambulate is worthwhile.

STANDING FRAMES

Most commercial standing frames are manufactured in sizes to fit children.[2] The geometry of a child with paraplegia differs from that of an adult with a comparable spinal cord disorder. As compared with adults, children are shorter, have a lower center of gravity, weigh less, and have proportionately larger feet in comparison with their height. Thus, less force is required to maintain upright posture, so the orthosis can be lighter and not as sturdy as one needed by an adult. An additional consideration may be that a child is more accustomed to being dressed and being told what to do. The concept of a wardrobe of orthoses suggests that as youngsters mature, they benefit from increasingly complex appliances.[3] Some standing orthoses are so stable that the child does not need to use crutches for additional support. Crutchless-standing frees the hands for exploring the environment. Orthoses thus foster the child's emotional, intellectual, and physical development. Unlike a table, which has an enclosure to support a child, the standing orthosis is more easily moved from place to place by a caregiver, enabling the youngster to play in different locations. Some well-coordinated children are able to move independently in a standing frame by leaning slightly to one side while rotating the upper trunk, then repeating the maneuver to the other side.

Unlike a custom-made trunk-hip-knee-ankle-foot orthosis, a standing frame does not have to fit precisely. The frame is not articulated, obviating the problem of placing orthotic joints in line with anatomic ones. Consequently, as the child grows taller, the same standing orthosis usually suffices. In addition, the standing frame does not have to be as sturdy as an articulated orthosis because it has no articulations.

"L" Standing Frame

The simplest standing frame resembles a capital "L" when viewed from the side (Figure 5-2). It consists of a broad wooden board approximately as long as the child is tall. A footboard is attached to the lower end of the main board. Chest and knee straps complete the frame. Sometimes casters are secured to the rear of the footboard so that the caregiver can roll the child from place to place. The "L" frame can be made easily. Commercially available "L" standing frames come in bright colors and even in the shape of animals (Figure 5-3).

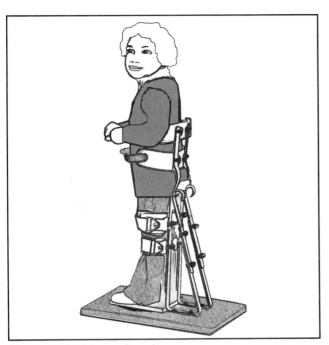

Figure 5-2. "L" standing frame.

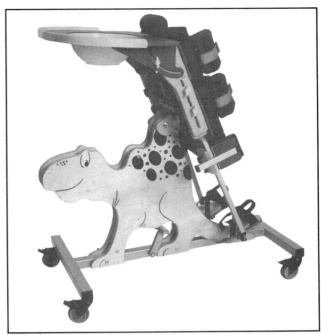

Figure 5-3. "L" standing frame in the shape of a dinosaur (reprinted with permission of Jenx Corporation).

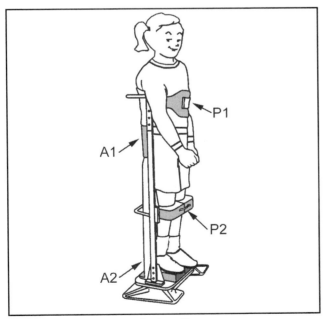

Figure 5-4. ORLAU swivel walker.

"A" Standing Frame

The "A" standing frame is more streamlined. It resembles a capital "A" when viewed from the back. The posterior support consists of two angled metal uprights with a transverse dorsolumbar band. The child's feet are strapped into footplates. The frame has a chest strap and a knee strap.

Swivel Walker

Another version of a standing frame was developed at the Orthotic Research and Locomotion Assessment Unit (ORLAU), Oswestry, England[4-6] (Figure 5-4). The posterior section is a curved aluminum or plastic trough, which facilitates donning. The swivel walker has the same type of chest and knee straps found in all standing frames. The footplate, however, is distinctive. Its upper surface has straps designed to secure the wearer's shoes. The lower surface has two swiveling plates, which facilitate ambulation. The plates slope upward and outward at a maximum angle of 6 degrees, permitting sideward rocking and enabling the opposite foot plate to clear the ground during ambulation. The swivel walker, unlike the other standing frames, is manufactured in both child and adult sizes. Patients can ambulate with it only on flat, smooth surfaces.

Parapodium

The parapodium (Figure 5-5) is an articulated version of a standing frame originated at the Ontario Crippled Children's Centre, now known as the Bloorview McMillan Centre, Toronto, Ontario, Canada. The orthosis has been refined at the University of Rochester in New York.[7] The aluminum orthosis has lateral uprights that terminate

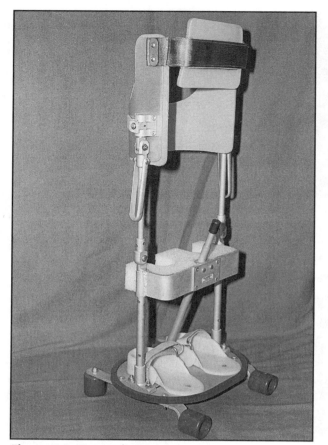

Figure 5-5. Parapodium.

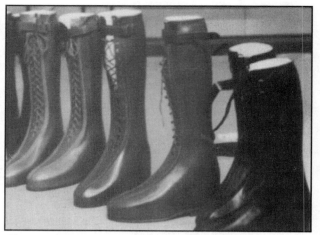

Figure 5-6a. Vannini-Rizzoli stabilizing ankle-foot orthosis.

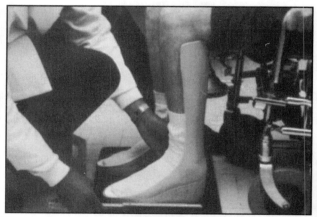

Figure 5-6b. Foot positioned in plantar flexion.

superiorly in a dorsolumbar band and inferiorly in a footplate with springs to secure the child's shoes. The orthosis has hip and knee joints that the child can operate by means of levers on each lateral upright. Chest and knee straps provide posteriorly directed force to keep the wearer upright. For sitting, the child can bend the orthotic hip and knee joints by rotating lateral levers bilaterally. To rise from a chair, the child either rotates the levers or pulls on a tele-scoping central rod that projects from the footplate. The Rochester version of parapodium also permits the wearer to retain the locked knees while flexing the hips, as when retrieving an object from the floor.

Any standing frame will enable the wearer to achieve stable standing. Those patients who have good coordination also learn to ambulate by shifting weight either to one edge of the "A" frame or para-podium or to one plate of the swivel walker. The individual then rotates the upper torso. The move-ment causes the wearer to rock onto the other edge or other footplate. The next step requires the individual to shift weight to the other plate, rocking on it. Movement is very stable and generally quite slow. A drawback of standing frames is that they cannot be worn under trousers.

Orthoses Designed for Ambulation

Ankle-Foot Orthoses: Vannini-Rizzoli Stabilizing Boots

A different orthotic approach for patients with paraplegia involves custom-made orthoses. The least encumbering orthoses are AFOs known as Vannini-Rizzoli stabilizing AFOs or boots (Figures 5-6a to 5-6c). Antoinetta Vannini, MD at the Rizzoli Institute in Bologna, Italy designed them. Intended for adults, each AFO features a flat shoe sole with the foot placed on a wedge. An essential element is an anteri-or strap located just below the knee. The strap

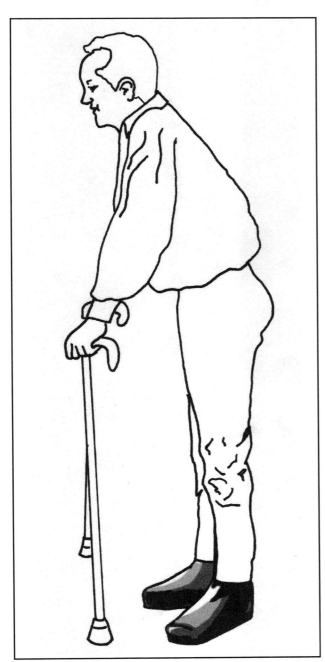

Figure 5-6c. On patient.

secures the leg against the posterior calf shell. One version of boot has an anterior leather component that has both laces and zippers. Initial adjustment is made with the laces. Subsequently, the wearer dons and doffs the device using the zippers.[8]

The boots prevent all foot and ankle motion. Knee and hip stabilization is achieved when the patient leans the torso backward. The iliofemoral ligaments limit hip hyperextension, while the knee capsules control knee hyperextension. People with spinal cord injury who have sensory loss at the level of the knee and below do not experience the discomfort that would otherwise be associated with the tendency to genu recurvatum. Absence of bracing over the knee makes sitting very easy. Ambulation requires the use of a walker or similar assistive device.

Stabilizing boots are contraindicated in the presence of hip or knee flexion contracture or marked spasticity or obesity.

Knee-Ankle-Foot Orthoses

Patients with lumbar lesions may manage with knee-ankle-foot orthoses (KAFOs). Whether the orthoses are AFO-SAs or have steel stirrups adjusted to limit motion, the speed of walking is not significantly different.[9]

Craig-Scott Orthoses

One of the most common orthotic designs for adults with paraplegia is known as the Craig-Scott KAFO.[10] They are named for the Craig Rehabilitation Center in Denver, Co, and Bruce Scott, the orthotist at the Craig Rehabilitation Center who designed them. Each leather-metal KAFO consists of a bichannel ankle lock stirrup riveted to a shoe that has a reinforced sole. The stirrup supports bilateral uprights, which support a locking knee joint and an anterior calf band. The uprights terminate at a thigh band and an anterior thigh strap. The distal portion of each KAFO may be either a metal stirrup (Figure 5-7a) or an AFO-SA (Figure 5-7b); the latter version (ie, the plastic KAFO) usually requires the use of high quarter shoes, but a sturdy low quarter shoe may suffice. Shock-absorbing inner or outer soles reduce the impact during walking.[11] Craig-Scott KAFOs are somewhat more expensive than other versions of KAFOs.[12]

Spreader Bar

Some patients have such severe adductor spasticity that their balance is precarious. They may find a steel spreader bar (Figure 5-8) attached to both medial uprights near the ankle to be a useful device. The bar prevents any hip adduction or rotation. It also limits the patient's ambulatory options to the swing-to or swing-through gaits, rather than the four- or two-point patterns.

Medially Linked KAFOs

A version of KAFOs for patients with juvenile and adult paraplegia was invented at the Royal North Shore Hospital, Sydney, Australia. Known as Walk-A-Bout or the Up and About (Figure 5-9), it has a ball-

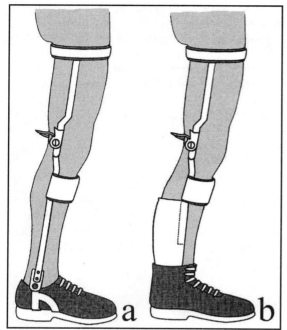

Figure 5-7. Craig-Scott KAFO. a. With steel stirrups. b. With a plastic solid ankle AFO.

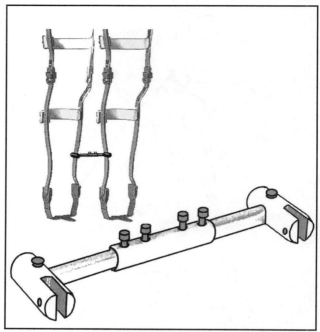

Figure 5-8. Spreader bar.

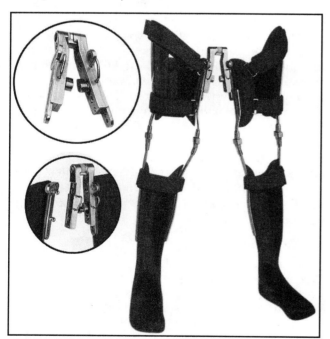

Figure 5-9. Medially linked KAFOs (photo provided courtesy of Cascade Orthopedic Supply).

bearing reciprocating linkage joining the proximal ends of the two medial uprights.[13-15] The linkage limits step length to the distance that the wearer can control. When the right leg is advanced, the left leg is prevented from flexing or extending unduly. Some

patients add a lumbosacral corset with inguinal straps to assist stability and leg control. The wearer must use crutches or similar assistive devices. Energy demand of ambulating with the Walk-A-Bout appears to be greater than that of the isocentric reciprocating gait orthosis, although rising and sitting are somewhat easier. A quick-release mechanism enables detaching the linkage, thus facilitating donning the orthosis.

As is the case with stabilizing boots, KAFOs are not suited to patients who have hip or knee flexion contracture, marked spasticity, or obesity.

Hip-Knee-Ankle-Foot Orthoses

Hip-knee-ankle-foot orthoses (HKAFOs) (Figures 5-10a and 5-10b) are sometimes prescribed for patients with paraplegia, particularly children born with spina bifida. The pelvic band with hip joints blocks hip abduction, adduction, and rotation. If drop ring locks are added to the hip joints, the orthosis also eliminates hip flexion and extension.

Trunk-Hip-Knee-Ankle-Foot Orthoses

Rigid THKAFO

The most conservative approach for adults and children with paraplegia is a custom-made trunk-hip-knee-ankle-foot orthosis (THKAFO) (Figures 5-11a and 5-11b). The device usually consists of a pair of plastic solid ankle orthoses and thigh shells with

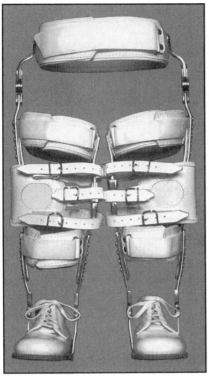

Figure 5-10a. HKAFO with bilateral uprights.

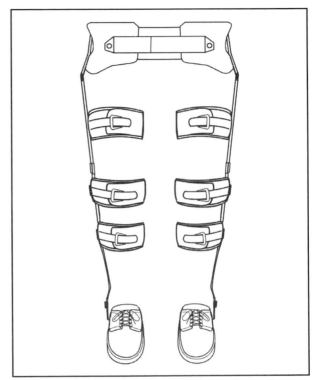

Figure 5-10b. Bilateral HKAFO with unilateral uprights.

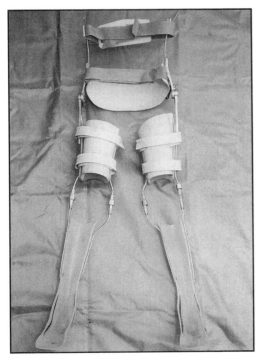

Figure 5-11a. THKAFO—anterior aspect.

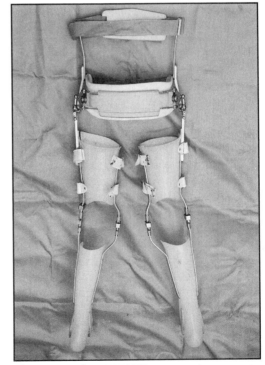

Figure 5-11b. THKAFO—posterior aspect.

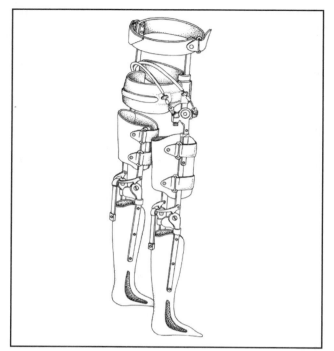

Figure 5-12. Reciprocating gait orthosis (reprinted with permission of Fillauer, Inc.).

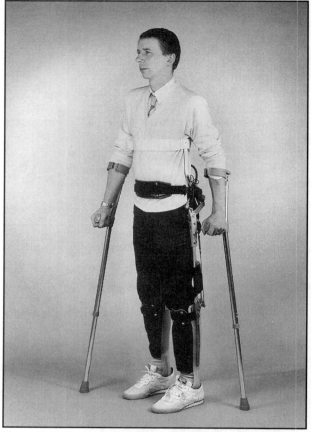

Figure 5-13. Advanced reciprocating gait orthosis (photo courtesy of H. Steeper Ltd. and Liberating Technologies).

lateral uprights, which incorporate locking knee joints and hip joints attached to a trunk orthosis. Some versions of THKAFO have bilateral uprights. When the patient stands with hips and knees locked, the THKAFO provides sufficient stability so that the wearer is unlikely to fall, assuming the person is supported by parallel bars or other assist. The hip joints restrict all hip motion so that any adductor spasticity cannot upset balance. A few well-coordinated and highly motivated patients learn to perform a swing-to or swing-through gait while wearing THKAFOs. Gait requires the use of parallel bars or crutches.

Although many patients are fitted with THKAFOs during their rehabilitation, long-term usage is minimal. The orthosis is very difficult to don, is relatively heavy, and does not provide any means of aiding leg motion needed for four-point ambulation. Moving to and from a chair is laborious. Other devices that provide the physiological and psychological benefits of standing, joint movement, and functional mobility are available.

Reciprocating Gait Orthoses

An articulated THKAFO may allow a child or adult with paraplegia to ambulate with a four- or two-point crutch gait. The reciprocating gait orthosis (RGO) (Figure 5-12) was invented at the Ontario Crippled Children's Centre and refined at Louisiana State University, New Orleans, La.[16-19] It consists of

a pair of KAFOs with solid ankles and locking knee joints. The RGO includes anterior leg and thigh straps. The KAFOs are attached to a pelvic band unit having hip joints, which permit only limited hip flexion and extension. Uprights that terminate in a rigid dorsal band and an anterior thoracic strap surmount the pelvic band.

The significant feature of RGOs is a steel cable or other assembly that joins the two hip joints and limits step length. When the wearer advances the right leg by rotating the torso, cable tension restrains flexion of the left leg. Consequently, during the double support phase of gait, the reciprocal link prevents bilateral hip collapse.[20] Once the individual shifts weight to the forwardly placed right leg, the wearer can advance the left leg. Gait is the relatively stable four- or two-point pattern, which requires a walker or similar assistive device.[21-26] A mechanism enables the wearer to unlock the hip and knee joints for sitting.

The advanced RGO (Figure 5-13) is a streamlined version designed for children and adults.[27,28] It has neither medial thigh uprights nor thigh cuffs; thus, it

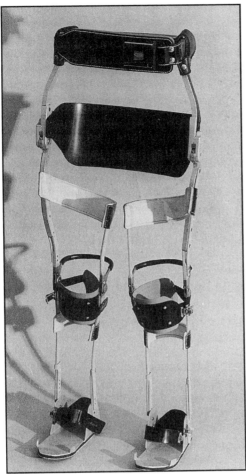

Figure 5-14. ParaWalker (reproduced from Jefferson RJ, Whittle MW. Performance of three walking orthoses: a case study using gait analysis. *Prosthet Orthot Int.* 1990;14:104 with permission of International Society for Prosthetics and Orthotics).

is an option. An adjustable assessment orthosis is available to enable evaluating patients before prescribing a custom-made appliance.

An alternative for children and adults is the isocentric RGO, which substitutes a centrally pivoting bar and tie rod arrangement for the original cable assembly. Lack of a cable reduces friction, increases durability, and presents a streamlined appearance.[29] An abduction hip joint is an option that increases frontal plane stability and eases perineal care. The physiologic cost index, obtained by dividing the difference between walking and resting heart rate by velocity, was lower with the isocentric RGO than with the basic RGO.[30-36] RGOs do not prevent progression of scoliosis in children who have been wearing them for several years.[37]

ParaWalker

A variation of the THKAFO developed in England is the ParaWalker[38,39] (Figure 5-14). It originated as the Hip Guidance Orthosis and was originally designed for children with spina bifida. The ParaWalker is the version fitted to adults with paraplegia.[40] Rather than having a cable joining the hips, the ParaWalker has exceptionally sturdy hip joints that have an adjustable feature, enabling the orthotist to determine the arc of hip motion. The orthosis has shoe plates with limited ankle motion joints to which the shoes are strapped and anterior leg bands. It is considerably heavier and more rigid than the RGO. As with other orthoses for paraplegia, the wearer needs an assistive device for ambulation.[41-44]

FUNCTIONAL ELECTRICAL STIMULATION

Some patients are interested in maintaining muscle tone so that joint mobility is preserved and sufficient soft tissue remains to prevent decubitus ulcers. These people may benefit from functional electrical stimulation, which involves application of a low-volt current to neural trigger points.[45-47] An electrical current causes muscular contractions, which prevent muscle fiber atrophy. Stationary bicycles and other exercise equipment have been adapted for use by patients with paraplegia who use functional electrical stimulation to achieve leg movement. A commercial application of functional electrical stimulation for ambulation is the ParaStep system (Sigmedics, Inc, Northfield, Ill).[48] Surface electrodes attached to the peroneal and femoral nerves enable the patient to achieve standing and slow ambulation. The system includes a walker that has a control module. The patient may select rise,

is less apt to interfere with perineal hygiene and donning. Patients can rise and sit more easily with this orthosis as compared with other RGOs because springs mounted in the thigh uprights assist hip extension during standing and control hip flexion during sitting. Knee-lock cables connect the hip and knee joints. Gas-filled struts provide knee extension force aid when standing. The patient leans forward until the knee-lock cables tighten to unlock the knee joints. Upper-limb force on a walker or other aid enables the individual to rise. As the hip joints straighten, the knees lock automatically. Rather than a steel cable, the advanced RGO has an efficient low-friction push/pull drive cable. A hip abduction lock

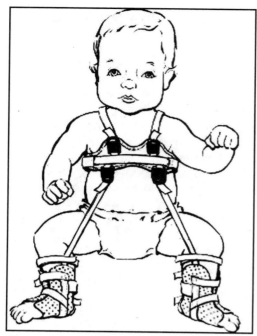

Figure 5-15. Pavlik harness.

walk, stop, and sit options. Some people have hybrid systems incorporating both functional electrical stimulation and orthoses.[49-54] The systems are expensive and fragile.

OTHER DEVICES FOR PARAPLEGIA

Regardless of orthosis, ambulation in the presence of thoracic paraplegia is slower and more arduous than normal walking. If the patient's primary concern is standing for physiological or emotional benefits or to extend the work area, then a standing frame is more economical and much easier to don than a custom-made orthosis for a child. An adult can achieve the same advantages by using a wheelchair equipped with a mechanism that converts the seat to a posterior support for standing.

FUNCTIONAL CONSIDERATIONS

Orthotic prescription for patients with paraplegia is influenced primarily by the level of the spinal cord lesion.[55] Longitudinal studies of children with spina bifida have confirmed that those with lesions below L3 continue ambulation during adulthood, provided they do not have marked contracture or obesity. Patients with higher lumbar lesions are less likely to persist with ambulation because they lack anatomical control of the knees.[56,57] AFOs and KAFOs are prescribed for patients with higher lumbar and thoracic lesions. Those with incomplete lesions are more likely to achieve orthotically assisted ambulation, especially in the household, and rely on the wheelchair for functional mobility. Ambulation, regardless of orthosis, is slower and more fatiguing than that of normal gait, with long periods of load transmission through the upper limbs.[58-60] The ability to don and doff the orthosis independently is a major determinant in long-term acceptance of the appliance.

The advent of alternatives to custom-made orthoses, such as standing frames, functional electrical stimulation, and standing wheelchairs, enables the rehabilitation team to make a more rational match between the patient's functional abilities and the most appropriate equipment.

HIP ORTHOSES

Hip Dislocation

Infants with congenital hip dislocation are often placed in an orthosis that maintains the femoral head in the acetabulum. The most popular of these devices is the Pavlik harness (Figure 5-15), a webbing chest harness with extensions to the feet. The physician adjusts buckles on the harness so that the hips are kept abducted, flexed, and externally rotated. The harness does not restrict the baby from kicking and moving about. It is washable and designed so that diaper changes are not hampered.

Legg-Calvé-Perthes Disease

Some youngsters develop chondroplastic disease of the femoral head. If left untreated, the head will deform into a characteristic mushroom configuration, which may lead to arthritic pain in early adulthood. Orthotic treatment (Figure 5-16a) is intended to keep the child ambulatory while protecting the femoral head as it goes through the degeneration and regeneration phases of the disease.

The more common approach is to permit weight bearing through the affected limb while protecting the hip. Two orthoses fulfill this purpose, namely the Atlanta (sometimes called Scottish Rite) and the Toronto orthoses. The Atlanta hip orthosis (HO) (Figure 5-16b) consists of a pelvic band and thigh cuffs. The cuffs are attached to the band by means of heavy metal hip joints, which restrict abduction, adduction, and rotation. The orthosis can be worn under clothing. The Toronto orthosis is more cumbersome. It has a pair of locked KAFOs joined by a bar at

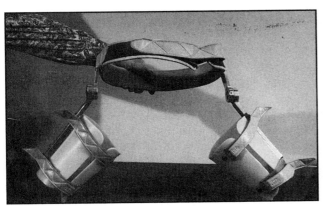

Figure 5-16a. Atlanta hip orthosis.

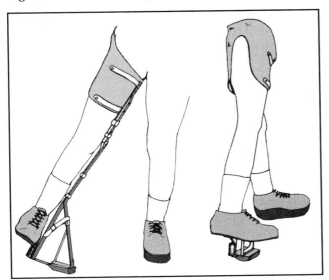

Figure 5-17. Trilateral orthosis.

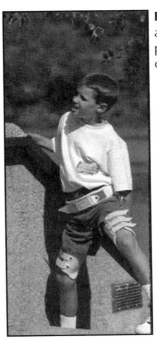

Figure 5-16b. Child wearing an Atlanta hip orthosis (reproduced with permission of Fillauer, Inc.).

the soles of the shoes. In the middle of the bar is a ball joint, which permits motion in all directions. The orthosis must be worn over trousers. The Toronto orthosis protects the wearer's knees while the Atlanta HO acts primarily at the hips.

Less common is the orthotic approach, which prevents weight-bearing through the affected limb. The trilateral orthosis (Figure 5-17) is a KAFO that has a thigh cuff, which is somewhat triangular in cross section. The distal lateral portion of the cuff is absent so that the orthosis applies no adducting force on the thigh. The uprights incorporate a locked knee joint. The distal end of the orthosis terminates in a patten, hoof-like platform. The shoe is placed laterally and is located so that no portion of the shoe touches the ground. The child must wear a contralateral shoe with a high lift so that the pelvis remains level.

All the orthotic approaches enable the child to walk without an assistive device.

Hip Control Orthoses

Children who have deficient hip control because of cerebral palsy or septic arthritis may benefit from a HO that restricts motion in one or more planes. The simplest such HO has a pelvic band to which two leg cuffs are joined by single-axis hinges. The HO permits hip flexion and extension but restricts motion in the frontal and transverse planes. For the nonambulatory child with a hip dislocation, a hip abduction KAFO (Figure 5-18) can hold the joint in place while healing occurs. A newer design is the Standing-Walking-and-Sitting-Hip (SWASH) Orthosis[61] (Figure 5-19). Its hinges permit sagittal motion and abduction.

Another way to control hip rotation involves fitting the child with a pair of KAFOs to which rotation-control straps are buckled[62] (Figure 5-20). To control internal rotation, two straps are secured to the posterior midline of a Dacron waist belt. The end of each strap is attached to the lateral upright of the KAFO. Tightening the straps causes the legs to rotate externally. To control external rotation, a Dacron strap is looped anteriorly from the right lateral upright to the left (Figure 5-21). Both the internal and the external rotation-control straps do not restrict frontal and sagittal hip motion and are less cumbersome than a rigid pelvic band with hip joints.

Postoperative Orthoses

Most orthotic manufacturers offer a range of HOs that limit the excursion of the hip joint in one or more

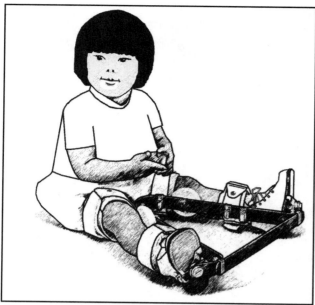

Figure 5-18. A hip abduction orthosis for nonambulatory children with hip dislocations.

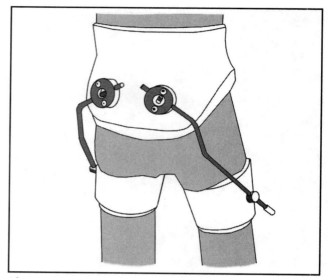

Figure 5-19. SWASH orthosis.

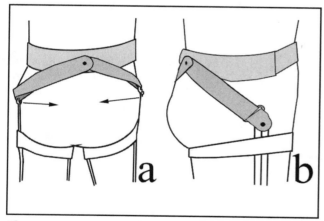

Figure 5-20. Internal rotation control straps. a. Posterior view. b. Sagittal view.

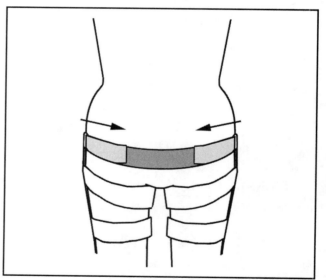

Figure 5-21. External rotation control straps, anterior view.

planes. The orthoses typically include a pelvic band and a thigh cuff. The hip joint has an adjustable mechanism, enabling the clinician to select the appropriate range of motion and to alter the excursion as necessary. These HOs are usually intended for adults who have had arthroplasty or similar surgery.

GUIDELINES FOR PRESCRIPTION

The following are biomechanical guidelines for prescribing orthoses for patients who have paraplegia:

1. To control hip flexion
   a. HKAFO with hip locks
2. To control hip rotation
   a. KAFOs with rotation-control straps
   b. KAFOs with a spreader bar
   c. HOs with single-axis hinges
   d. SWASH orthosis
   e. HKAFO with or without hip locks
3. To stabilize paralyzed hips, knees, and ankles
   a. Standing frame
   b. Parapodium
   c. Swivel walker
   d. Vannini-Rizzoli Stabilizing AFOs

e. Craig-Scott KAFOs
f. Medially linked KAFOs
g. Reciprocating gait orthosis
h. ParaWalker/hip guidance orthosis

Guidelines for prescribing orthoses for patients who have hip disease or who lack hip control include the following:

1. To promote resolution of congenital hip dislocation in infants
   a. Pavlik harness
2. To preserve femoral head convexity in the presence of Legg-Calvé-Perthes disease
   a. Atlanta HO
   b. Toronto KAFO
   c. Trilateral KAFO
3. To restrict a child's hip motion in one or more planes
   a. HO with single-axis hip joints
   b. SWASH orthosis
   c. KAFOs with rotation-control straps
   d. HKAFO with hip joints with or without locks
   e. THKAFO with hip joints with or without locks
4. To restrict an adult's hip motion in one or more planes
   a. HO with adjustable hinges

SUMMARY

Children and adults with paraplegia, whether caused by spinal cord injury, congenital malformation, or other factors, may be provided with orthoses that enable them to stand. The standing frame, parapodium, and swivel walker all include a foot platform and utilize a four-point system to stabilize the wearer, namely posteriorly directed forces from chest and knee bands and anteriorly directed forces from a dorsolumbar bar and the shoes. Some individuals learn to shift weight to one edge of the foot platform to ambulate by exaggerated motion of the upper torso. Orthoses designed to facilitate walking include some mode of stabilizing the ankle and foot. AFOs align the lower limbs so that the axes of the knees and hips are posterior to the weight line. KAFOs provide orthotic stabilization of the feet and knees, but they also require hips to be aligned behind the weight line. THKAFOs include rigid braces, various designs of reciprocating gait orthosis, and the ParaWalker, all of which enable the agile person to ambulate slowly at substantial energy cost.

Alternatives to orthoses for standing and walking are functional electrical stimulation systems and wheelchairs with standing mechanisms.

Hip orthoses are designed for infants with dislocated hips, youngsters with Legg-Calvé-Perthes disease, and adults with hip arthroplasty.

THOUGHT QUESTIONS

1. For a 6-year-old boy with Legg-Calvé-Perthes disease in the left hip, under what circumstances would you recommend a KO, an Atlanta HO, or a trilateral KAFO?
2. Diagram the ground reaction force vectors throughout the stance phase for a patient wearing Craig-Scott KAFOs. Include forces at the pelvis, hips, knees, ankles, and feet.
3. Diagram the ground reaction force vectors throughout the stance phase for a patient wearing Vannini-Rizzoli AFOs. Include forces at the pelvis, hips, knees, ankles, and feet. How does your response to this question compare with your response to the previous question?
4. Many orthoses are provided for people with high-level paraplegia during their rehabilitation, even though such individuals are unlikely to become functional ambulators. Should all patients with paraplegia have orthoses if they request them, even when their goals for functional ambulation are unrealistic? Take a position on this issue and justify it.

REFERENCES

1. Cybulski GR, Jaeger RJ. Standing performance of persons with paraplegia. *Arch Phys Med Rehabil.* 1986;67:103-108.
2. Edelstein JE. Orthotic options for standing and walking. *Topics in Spinal Cord Injury Rehabilitation.* 2000;5:11-23.
3. Ryan KD, Ploski C, Emans JB. Myelodysplasia—the musculoskeletal problem: habilitation from infancy to adulthood. *Phys Ther.* 1991;71:935-946.
4. Major RE, Stallard J, Farmer SE. A review of 42 patients of 16 years and over using the ORLAU ParaWalker. *Prosthet Orthot Int.* 1997;21:147-152.
5. Stallard J, Farmer IR, Poiner R, et al. Engineering design considerations of the ORLAU swivel walker. *Engineering Medicine.* 1986;15:3-7.
6. Stallard J, Henshaw JH, Lomas B, Poiner R. The ORLAU VCG (variable centre of gravity) swivel walker for muscular dystrophy patients. *Prosthet Orthot Int.* 1992;16:46-48.
7. Gram M, Kinnen E, Brown JA. Parapodium redesigned for sitting. *Phys Ther.* 1981;61:657-660.

8. Kent HO. Vannini-Rizzoli stabilizing orthosis (boot): preliminary report on a new ambulatory aid for spinal cord injury. *Arch Phys Med Rehabil.* 1992;73:302-307.

9. Krebs DE, Edelstein JE, Fishman S. Comparison of plastic/metal and leather/metal knee-ankle-foot orthoses. *Am J Phys Med Rehabil.* 1988;67:175-185.

10. Scott BA. Engineering principles and fabrication techniques for the Scott-Craig long-leg brace for paraplegics. *Orthotics and Prosthetics.* 1971;25:14-19.

11. Bierling-Sorensen F, Ryde H, Boisen-Moller F, Lyquist E. Shock absorbing material on the shoes of long leg braces for paraplegic walking. *Prosthet Orthot Int.* 1990;14:27-32.

12. Atrice MB. Lower extremity orthotic management for the spinal-cord-injured client. *Topics in Spinal Cord Injury Rehabilitation.* 2000;5:1-10.

13. Middleton JW, Fisher W, Davis GM, Smith RM. A medial linkage orthosis to assist ambulation after spinal cord injury. *Prosthet Orthot Int.* 1998;23:258-264.

14. Middleton JW, Sinclair PJ, Smith RM, Davis GM. Postural control during stance in paraplegia: effects of medially linked versus unlinked knee-ankle-foot orthoses. *Arch Phys Med Rehabil.* 1999;80:1558-1565.

15. Saitoh E, Suzuki T, Sonoda S, et al. Clinical experience with a new hip-knee-foot orthotic system using a medial single hip joint for paraplegic standing and walking. *Am J Phys Med Rehabil.* 1996;75:198-203.

16. Beckman J. The Louisiana State University reciprocating gait orthosis. *Physiotherapy.* 1987;73:386-392.

17. Douglas R, Larson PF, D'Ambrosia R, McCall RE. The LSU reciprocation-gait orthosis. *Orthopedics.* 1983;6:834-839.

18. Jaeger RJ, Yarkony GM, Roth EJ. Rehabilitation technology for standing and walking after spinal cord injury. *Am J Phys Med Rehabil.* 1989;68:128-133.

19. Phillips DL, Field RE, Broughton NS, Menelaus MB. Reciprocating orthoses for children with myelomeningocele. *J Bone Joint Surg [Br].* 1995;77:110-113.

20. Dall P, Granat M. The function of the reciprocal link in paraplegic orthotic gait. *Journal of Prosthetics and Orthotics.* 2001;13:10-13.

21. Bernardi M, Canale I, Castellano Y, et al. The efficiency of walking of paraplegic patients using a reciprocating gait orthosis. *Paraplegia.* 1995;33:409-415.

22. Crosbie WJ, Nichol AC. Reciprocal aided gait in paraplegia. *Paraplegia.* 1990;28:353-363.

23. Ekus L, McHugh L. A new look at the RGO protocol. *Clinical Prosthetics and Orthotics.* 1987;11:79-81.

24. Guidera KJ, Smith S, Raney E, et al. Use of the reciprocating gait orthosis in myelodysplasia. *J Pediatr Orthop.* 1993;13:341-348.

25. Knutson LM, Clark DE. Orthotic devices for ambulation in children with cerebral palsy and myelomeningocele. *Phys Ther.* 1991;71:947-960.

26. Lotta S, Fiocchi A, Giovannini R, et al. Restoration of gait with orthoses in thoracic paraplegia: a multicenter investigation. *Paraplegia.* 1994;32:608-615.

27. Baardman G, Ijzerman MJ, Hermens HJ, et al. The influence of the reciprocal hip joint link in the advanced reciprocating gait orthosis on standing performance in paraplegia. *Prosthet Orthot Int.* 1997;21:210-221.

28. Ijzerman MJ, Baardman G, Hermens HJ, et al. The influence of the reciprocal cable in the advanced reciprocating gait orthosis on paraplegic gait performance. *Prosthet Orthot Int.* 1997;21:52-61.

29. Campbell JH. Reciprocating gait orthosis with linear bearing. *Journal of the Association of Children's Prosthetic/Orthotic Clinics.* 1990;25:2-5.

30. Franceschini M, Barata S, Zampolini M, et al. Reciprocating gait orthoses: a multicenter study of their use by spinal cord injured patients. *Arch Phys Med Rehabil.* 1997;78:582-586.

31. Harvey LA, Davis GM, Smith MB, Engel S. Energy expenditure during gait using the Walk-A-Bout and isocentric reciprocal gait orthoses in persons with paraplegia. *Arch Phys Med Rehabil.* 1998;79:945-949.

32. Harvey LA, Smith MB, Davis GM, Engel S. Functional outcomes attained by T9-12 paraplegic patients with the Walk-A-Bout and the isocentric reciprocal gait orthoses. *Arch Phys Med Rehabil.* 1997;78:706-711.

33. Ijzerman MJ, Baardman G, Hermens HJ, et al. Comparative trials on hybrid walking systems for people with paraplegia: an analysis of study methodology. *Prosthet Orthot Int.* 1999;23:260-273.

34. Jefferson RJ, Whittle MW. Performance of three walking orthoses for the paralyzed: a case study gait analysis. *Prosthet Orthot Int.* 1990;14:103-110.

35. Kelly M. Swivel walker vs. parapodium vs. reciprocal gait orthoses in children and adolescents with spinal cord injuries. *Phys Ther.* 1991;71:S8. Abstract.

36. McCall RE, Schmidt WT. Clinical experience with the reciprocal gait orthosis in myelodysplasia. *J Pediatr Orthop.* 1986;6:157-161.

37. Campbell JH. Outcome study: the progression of spinal deformity in paraplegic children fitted with reciprocating gait orthoses. *Prosthet Orthot Int.* 1999;11:79-84.

38. Butler PB, Major R. The ParaWalker: a rational approach to the provision of reciprocal ambulation for paraplegic patients. *Physiotherapy.* 1987;73:393-397.

39. Butler PB, Major RE, Patrick JH. The technique of reciprocal walking using the hip guidance orthosis (HGO) with crutches. *Prosthet Orthot Int.* 1984;8:33-38.

40. Moore P, Stallard J. A clinical review of adult paraplegic patients with complete lesion using the ORLAU ParaWalker. *Paraplegia.* 1991;29:191-196.

41. Nene AV, Jennings SJ. Physiological cost index of paraplegic locomotion using the ORLAU ParaWalker. *Paraplegia.* 1992;30:246-252.

42. Nene AV, Major RE. Dynamics of reciprocal gait of adult paraplegics using the ParaWalker (hip guidance orthosis). *Prosthet Orthot Int.* 1987;11:124-127.

43. Nene AV, Patrick JH. Energy cost of paraplegic locomotion with the ORLAU ParaWalker. *Paraplegia.* 1989;27:5-15.

44. Patrick JH, McClelland MR. Low energy cost reciprocal walking for the adult paraplegic. *Paraplegia.* 1985;23:113-117.

45. Bajd Y, Kralj A, Turk H, et al. Use of functional electrical stimulation in the rehabilitation of patients with incomplete spinal cord injuries. *Journal of Biomedical Engineering.* 1989;11:96-102.

46. Bonaroti D, Akers JM, Smith BT, et al. Comparison of functional electrical stimulation to long leg braces for upright mobility for children with complete thoracic level spinal injuries. *Arch Phys Med Rehabil.* 1999;80:1047-1053.

47. Granat M, Keating JF, Smith AC, et al. The use of functional electrical stimulation to assist gait in patients with incomplete spinal cord injury: observed benefits during gait studies. *Paraplegia.* 1993;31:207-215.

48. Claiborne EG, Baxter KK. Introduction to the ParaStep system. *Neurology Report.* 1994;18:11-12.

49. Hirokawa S, Grimm M, Le T, et al. Energy consumption in paraplegic ambulation using the reciprocating gait orthosis and electrical stimulation of the thigh muscles. *Arch Phys Med Rehabil.* 1990;71:687-694.

50. Isakov E, Douglas R, Berns P. Ambulation using the reciprocal gait orthosis and functional electrical stimulation. *Paraplegia.* 1992;30:239-245.

51. McClelland MR, Andrews BJ, Patrick JH, et al. Augmentation of the Oswestry ParaWalker by means of surface electrical stimulation gait analysis of three patients. *Paraplegia.* 1987;25:32-38.

52. Petrofsky JS, Smith JB. Physiologic costs of computer-controlled walking in persons with paraplegia using a reciprocating-gait orthosis. *Arch Phys Med Rehabil.* 1991;72:890-896.

53. Phillips CA. Electrical muscle stimulation in combination with a reciprocating gait orthosis for ambulation by paraplegics. *Journal of Biomedical Engineering.* 1989;11:338-344.

54. Phillips CA, Hendershot DM. Functional electrical stimulation and reciprocating gait orthosis for ambulation exercise in a tetraplegic patient: a case study. *Paraplegia.* 1991;29:268-276.

55. Barbeau H, Ladouceur M, Norman KE, et al. Walking after spinal cord injury: evaluation, treatment, and functional recovery. *Arch Phys Med Rehabil.* 1999;80:225-235.

56. Flandry F, Burke S, Roberts J, et al. Functional ambulation in myelodysplasia: the effect of orthotic selection on physical and physiologic performance. *J Pediatr Orthop.* 1986;6:661-665.

57. Solomonow M. Performance of walking orthosis for paraplegics. *Gait Posture.* 1995;3:86. Abstract.

58. Bowker P, Messenger N, Ogilvie C, Rowley DI. Energetics of paraplegic walking. *J Biomed Eng.* 1992;14:344-350.

59. Miller NE, Merritt JL, Merkel KD, Westbrook PR. Paraplegic energy expenditure during negotiation of architectural barriers. *Arch Phys Med Rehabil.* 1984;65:778-779.

60. Nene AV, Hermens HJ, Zilvold G. Paraplegic locomotion: a review. *Spinal Cord.* 1996;34:507-524.

61. Torpey PC, Herrle SE. Use of the S.W.A.S.H. orthosis for sitting and gait function in a child with sequelae of septic hip. *Physical Therapy Case Reports.* 2000;45-56.

62. Hoffman E. Hip-rotation control straps. *Inter-Clinic Informatin Bulletin.* 1983;18:1-4.

RECOMMENDED READING

1. Solomonow M, Baratta R, D'Ambrosia R. Standing and walking after spinal cord injury: experience with the reciprocating gait orthosis powered by electrical muscle stimulation. *Topics in Spinal Cord Injury Rehabilitation.* 2000;5:29-53.

2. Stallard J, Major RE. The influence of orthosis stiffness on paraplegic ambulation and its implications for functional electrical stimulation (FES) walking systems. *Prosthet Orthot Int.* 1995;19:108-114.

3. Stallard J, Major RE. A review of reciprocal walking systems for paraplegic patients: factors affecting choice and economic justification. *Prosthet Orthot Int.* 1998;22:240-247.

4. Stallard J, Major RE, Butler PB. The orthotic ambulatory performance of paraplegic myelomeningocele children using the ORLAU ParaWalker treatment system. *Clin Rehabil.* 1991;5:111-114.

5. Stallard J, Patrick JH, Major RE. A review of the fundamental design problems of providing ambulation for paraplegic patients. *Paraplegia.* 1989;27:70-75.

6. Stein RB, Belanger M, Wheeler G, et al. Electrical systems for improving locomotion after incomplete spinal cord injury: an assessment. *Arch Phys Med Rehabil.* 1993;74:954-959.

7. Strachan RK, Cook J, Wilkie W, Kennedy NSJ. An evaluation of pneumatic orthoses in thoracic paraplegia. *Paraplegia.* 1985;23:295-305.

8. Summers BN, McClelland MR, El Masri WS. A clinical review of the adult hip guidance orthosis (ParaWalker) in traumatic paraplegics. *Paraplegia.* 1988;26:19-26.

9. Sykes L, Edwards J, Powell ES, Ross RS. The reciprocating gait orthosis: long-term usage patterns. *Arch Phys Med Rehabil.* 1995;76:779-783.

10. Sykes L, Ross RS, Powell ES, Edwards J. Objective measurement of use of the reciprocating gait orthosis (RGO) and the electrically augmented RGO in adult patients with spinal cord lesions. *Prosthet Orthot Int.* 1996;20:182-190.

11. Thoume P, Perrouin-Verbe P, LeClaire G, et al. Restoration of functional gait in paraplegic patients with the RGO-II hybrid orthosis. *Paraplegia.* 1995;33:647-653.

12. Vazquez MA. The use of Intrathecal Lioresal pump and reciprocating gait orthosis for functional gait in spastic paraparesis in an adult: a case report. *Arch Phys Med Rehabil.* 1996;77:986. Abstract.

13. Watkins EM, Edwards DE, Patrick JH. ParaWalker paraplegic walking. *Physiotherapy.* 1987;73:99-100.

14. Whittle MW. Paraplegic locomotion. *Clin Rehabil.* 1988;2:45-49.

15. Whittle MW, Cochrane GM, Chase AP, et al. A comparative trial of two walking systems for paralyzed people. *Paraplegia.* 1991;29:97-102.

16. Winchester PK, Carollo JJ, Parekh RN, et al. A comparison of paraplegic gait performance using two types of reciprocating gait orthoses. *Prosthet Orthot Int.* 1993;17:101-106.

17. Yano H, Kaneko S, Nakazawa K, et al. A new concept of dynamic orthosis for paraplegia: the weight bearing control (WBC) orthosis. *Prosthet Orthot Int.* 1997;21:222-228.

CASE STUDIES

For the following cases, select an appropriate orthosis, establish long- and short-term treatment goals, and develop a treatment plan.

- CR is a 45-year-old high school teacher who was struck by a car while crossing the street. She sustained an incomplete L2 spinal cord lesion. Clonus is present in both Achilles' tendons, with the right greater than the left. She has no sensation below the level of the lesion. She has no joint contractures. All muscles above the level of the lesion have normal strength. Muscle test grades for other muscles bilaterally are iliopsoas, poor; quadratus lumborum, good; lumbar extensors, fair; all other lower-limb muscles, zero.

- PD is a 3-year-old boy with spina bifida at the L3 level, mild hydrocephalus, and an IQ of 90. During his first year, he had four open-heart surgical procedures to correct a congenital defect, and he could not be placed prone because of the surgical incisions and drainage tubes. He developed head control at 27 months and independent circle sitting at 30 months. He can now creep reciprocally, pull to stand, and is beginning to cruise along furniture.

- DC is a 25-year-old man who sustained a complete T12 spinal cord lesion when he lost control of his motorcycle and crashed into a tree at 85 mph. He had spinal fusion, skeletal traction, and was in a coma for 2 weeks. When he regained consciousness he had no sensation below the groin and no recollection of the accident. He left high school in the middle of his junior year and had been a seasonal construction worker. He has a history of alcoholism. He has been verbally abusive to the rehabilitation staff at the spinal cord unit and has refused to participate in the exercise program. His psychologist reports that he has expressed suicidal thoughts.

- FH was born with congenital hip dislocation secondary to shallow acetabula, bilaterally. She is 3 months old.

- MC is a 6-year-old boy who has just been diagnosed with Legg-Calvé-Perthes disease. He complains of severe pain in his left hip that sometimes radiates to his groin and along the left thigh. He walks with lateral trunk bending to the left and has point tenderness of the left hip. He has difficulty running, walking on a balance beam, and maintaining balance in single-limb standing on the left leg. Radiographs confirm avascular necrosis of the left femoral head.

- NS is an 84-year-old woman with severe osteoarthritis of the left hip. During left stance phase, she has marked lean to the left. She has a positive Trendelenburg's sign when standing on the left leg. She lives alone on the second floor of an apartment house that has no elevator. She has increasing difficulty negotiating the flight of stairs and has an especially difficult time carrying groceries. The pain in her left hip is getting worse, and she is now starting to experience low back pain.

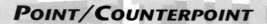

POINT/COUNTERPOINT

EL is a 12-year-old girl with spina bifida at L3-4. Quadriceps motor power is fair bilaterally. She is overweight and does not participate in physical activity. She has dull normal intelligence. Feet exhibit pes calcaneus, insensitivity, and edema bilaterally.

JOAN SAYS	JAN SAYS

Orthotic Prescription

She seems to be unwilling to cope with orthoses. Consequently, I recommend the simplest bracing. Elastic hose would control edema and shield her insensitive skin from edge pressure from an orthosis. She should be able to achieve knee and foot control with a pair of AFO-SAs with anterior bands. The shoe inserts should be contoured to apply total contact to plantar surfaces of her feet. Her shoes should have resilient heels and rocker bars to aid early and late stance, respectively.

I would like to use the least extensive bracing that would permit her to ambulate because I am concerned about her willingness to wear any type of orthosis. She should wear elastic hose to control edema. She would benefit from bilateral plastic AFO-SAs decorated with cartoons and in the color of her choice. Canvas tennis shoes with rocker bars will facilitate momentum during stance phase.

Long-Term Goals

- Increase duration of ambulation
- Peer group (eg, Girl Scouts or Special Olympics) to increase physical activity and improve self-esteem

- Self-inspection of skin
- Foot hygiene
- Household ambulation
- Wheelchair use in the community
- Peer group to help her maintain weight control and improve self-image
- Eventually, driver's education to operate automobile with hand controls

Short-Term Goals

- Independent donning
- Self-inspection of skin
- Household ambulation without cane; community ambulation with one or two canes

- Don and doff orthoses independently
- Care for the orthoses
- Wheelchair mobility
- Manage edema with massage, elevation, and elastic hose

Physical Therapy Plan

- Instruct patient in donning and skin inspection
- Gait training with and without cane(s)
- Referral to peer group

- Patient education
  a. Don and doff orthoses and care for them
  b. Self-inspection of skin
  c. Foot hygiene
  d. Foot massage
- Wheelchair transfers and mobility
- Gait training for household ambulation
- Referral to peer-support group

Chapter 6

Evaluation Procedures for Lower-Limb Orthoses

"I can tell where my own shoe pinches me."
Miguel de Cervantes, *Don Quixote*

Thoughtful prescription and individualized training involve the patient's having an orthosis that fits and functions properly. An orthosis that is not well constructed may be less attractive and is likely to injure the patient and malfunction prematurely. Consequently, orthotic evaluation is an essential part of rehabilitation. This chapter details evaluation procedures for lower-limb orthoses as well as directions for caring for the full range of orthoses, both custom-made and mass-produced. Evaluation procedures for trunk and cervical orthoses appear in Chapter 7 and for upper-limb orthoses in Chapter 8.

ADMINISTRATIVE CONSIDERATIONS

The orthosis should be evaluated when it is delivered to the patient and before the individual wears it on a regular basis. Deficiencies in fit, mechanical componentry, or construction should be identified and corrected; otherwise, the patient risks developing skin irritation or faulty postural or gait habits to compensate for orthotic inadequacies. An appliance that presses on sensitive structures may also cause the patient to refuse to wear it.

The orthosis should be reevaluated when the patient is about to be discharged or transferred to another treatment setting. At this point, the individual has worn it for several weeks and incipient deficiencies may become apparent. These problems should be corrected before the patient leaves the close supervision of the rehabilitation department. Discharge planning should include scheduling the reevaluation of the patient's function, including the adequacy of the orthosis. Because children grow, reevaluation of their orthoses should occur at least every 3 months. Provision for longitudinal and circumferential adjustment in pediatric orthoses is important.

The professional members of the core clinic team, namely the orthotist, the physical therapist, and the physician, should conduct the evaluation and subsequent reevaluation in consultation with the patient. In a busy clinic, it is often the physical therapist who conducts a detailed assessment then presents key conclusions to the team. Ordinarily, the orthotist also inspects the device thoroughly before delivering it.

At the time of delivery, the team may decide that the orthosis is entirely satisfactory and the patient may proceed to wear it. Alternatively, the team may identify minor problems that would not jeopardize the patient's skin or balance yet should be rectified prior to discharge. Again, the patient can embark on a wearing program. The third consequence of the initial evaluation is that one or more major deficiencies are evident. In such circumstances, the patient should not wear the orthosis until corrections are made. For example, a shoe that does not fit properly will compel the wearer to limit weight-bearing and adopt other undesirable compensations.

Evaluation of the adequacy of a particular orthosis for a given patient involves a static and a dynamic examination. Static evaluation consists of observing the orthosis on the patient as the individual stands and sits, as well as examining the device off the patient. Dynamic evaluation is performed while the patient walks.

STATIC EVALUATION

Prior to assisting the patient into the orthosis, team members should check that it conforms with the prescription.

Considerations for All Orthoses

The patient's opinion regarding whether the orthosis has satisfactory weight, comfort, function, and appearance is paramount. A person who is keenly distressed about the appearance of the orthosis will not wear it even if the orthosis meets all objective standards. The patient is the only individual who can judge the comfort of the orthosis, regardless of whether or not the clinic team is satisfied with the contour and alignment of the appliance. Sometimes peer support can help the patient understand the characteristics of the orthosis. Conversely, the patient may be pleased with an orthosis that the clinic team judges to be substandard. In such an instance, it is important to retain the patient's confidence in the orthosis while making required changes in fit, alignment, or construction.

A critical aspect of evaluation is the ease in which the patient is able to don the orthosis. At the time of delivery, one can expect that the individual may be unfamiliar with the donning procedure and needs assistance. If, for example, the patient has hemiplegia and perceptual deficit, then a laced shoe would probably remain difficult to manage. Ordinarily, the clinic team would have realized the need for specifying pressure-sensitive tape shoe closures in place of laces. If, for any reason, the shoes arrive with laces, then the closure should be altered so that the patient can regain self-sufficiency. Clearly, an orthosis that is too snug will be difficult, if not impossible, to don and must be modified or a new one provided.

The patient must be able to sit comfortably in an unupholstered straight chair with hips, knees, and ankles at approximately 90 degrees while wearing the orthosis. Comfort in sitting requires that the calf band not encroach into the popliteal fossa. A sharp superior margin of the calf band compromises sitting comfort. With a KAFO, the proximal margin of the calf band and the distal margin of the distal thigh band should be equidistant from the orthotic joint axis to minimize the risk of soft tissue being squeezed posteriorly. The orthotic knee axis should lie in the vicinity of the anatomic knee axis, slightly above the tibial plateau. Too low or too high an axis interferes with knee flexion and extension. Too tight a knee pad in a KAFO also makes sitting uncomfortable.

Prior to applying the orthosis, one should inspect the patient's skin, noting any scars, blemishes, or other discolorations. At the conclusion of the static and dynamic evaluation, the orthosis should be removed so that the team can evaluate the construction of the orthosis. During the time it takes to examine the orthosis, the patient should be resting. Any skin induration, blanching, or redness should subside within 10 minutes. Otherwise, one can conclude that the orthosis is too tight and must be adjusted. Mechanical joints or uprights that press on the skin will eventually irritate the skin and may lead to ulceration.

The clinic team should examine the construction of the device, paying particular attention to smoothness of edges and interior and exterior surfaces. A sharp brim may impinge on soft tissue, especially if the patient is obese. Interior roughness, such as that caused by protruding rivets or other metal fixtures, can abrade the skin, while a rough exterior may damage overlying clothing. Shoe modifications should blend smoothly with the rest of the shoe. A stirrup should be riveted to the shoe so that the shoe interior does not have protruding rivet heads. Plastic components should be molded with uniform thickness with no indications of excessive heat, which might lead to failure. Lamination should be uniform with no areas in which the resin has not penetrated the fabric matrix. Screws and rivets should lie flat on the surface of uprights. Hammer nicks and excessively sharp bends are sites for stress concentration, which may lead to breakage. Straps should be well secured with the edges neatly finished and with sufficient material so that the orthosis may be subsequently tightened or loosened. Leather should be sewn with uniform stitches with thread ends secured. Knee and hip locks and other mechanisms should operate easily and securely.

Shoe Inspection

- Ball of the shoe (widest part of the sole) lies at the ball of the foot (metatarsophalangeal joints)
- Shoe is 1 cm longer than the foot
- Heel counter hugs the posterior heel
- Toe box covers the dorsum comfortably
- Provision for adjusting to increased foot volume during the day
- Foot is well supported medially and laterally
- Shoe insert lodges snugly in the shoe

Regardless of its purpose, the shoe should fit properly after all modifications are complete and any insert is installed. Shoe size is an inadequate guide to shoe fit. When assessing shoe fit, check each foot separately. Ideally, shoe fit should be examined at the end of the day when any swelling will be at a maximum. The shoe should feel comfortable as soon as it is donned; expecting that an uncomfortable shoe will "break in" is fallacious. Shoe fit should be judged when the wearer is standing. Weight-bearing stresses the ligaments of the foot, elongating and widening the foot. The shoe should be 1 cm longer than the longest toe and should be as wide as the metatarsophalangeal width of the foot. A short shoe will interfere with toe action in late stance and will force the toes into hammer toe deformity. An overly long shoe may cause the wearer to trip at late stance; in addition, the contours of the excessively long shoe will not match the shape of the foot, particularly at the metatarsophalangeal region. A shoe that is too wide will allow the foot to slide and will eventually cause blisters; a narrow shoe interferes with the metatarsophalangeal hyperextension that is essential in late stance. The counter, the reinforcement of the posterior part of the shoe, should fit snugly without undue gapping. Too loose a counter will interfere with late stance and may induce a blister. A tight counter will be painful or may cause a pressure sore. A low shoe should be shaped so that the upper does not irritate either malleolus; consequently, the lateral side should be cut lower than the medial side.

The toe box should cover the dorsum without impinging on hammer toes or claw toes if present. The shoe should have some provision for accommodating changes in foot volume during the day; lacing provides greatest adjustability but may be difficult for the patient to manipulate. If so, then the shoe should have several straps. The shoe should support the foot medially and laterally. This criterion is difficult to meet in the presence of severe spasticity or obesity. An insert should fit both the foot and the shoe. Patients should be informed of the necessity of using the insert only in shoes that have the same design and last type, rather than indiscriminately switching between low- and higher-heeled shoes.

The shoe that the patient has worn for several weeks or longer is an important source of information regarding the patient's habitual loading pattern. A shoe that does not match the size and shape of the wearer's foot will exhibit distortion of the upper. For example, if the toe box is excessively narrow, the upper will show erosion in the vicinity of the fifth toe, the hallux, or on both sides. A medially bulged upper indicates pes planus. Scuffing of the distal end of the shoe occurs when the wearer drags the foot, perhaps in response to weakness of the dorsiflexors. Erosion of the inside of the counter is caused by excessive heel motion and indicates that the counter is too loose. On the sole, a wear pattern confined to the longitudinal midline results when the shoe is too narrow. Excessive erosion on the lateral border of the sole suggests pes varus. Normally, the posterolateral border of the heel is eroded more than any other part of the heel. Noticeable wear elsewhere on the heel indicates abnormal foot posture.

One should also compare the left shoe with the right. Asymmetrical erosion can be caused by leg- or foot-length discrepancy, anatomical variation, or neurological deficit.

Ankle-Foot Orthosis Inspection

- Shell or calf band is comfortable
- Shell or uprights conform to the contour of the leg
- Fibular head sustains minimal or no pressure
- Mechanical ankle joints coincide with the anatomical ankle
- Varus or valgus correction strap supports the foot
- Patellar tendon-bearing brim reduces weight-bearing at the heel

When the pressure that the orthosis applies to the body is tolerable, the patient is likely to be comfortable. Bands and shells should apply uniform contact to the skin, rather than concentrate pressure on a small area. A plastic band or shell should be molded to conform to the shape of the patient's leg. Bands should apply equal pressure at their upper and lower margins. In an adult's orthosis, a calf band that is less than 8 cm wide is apt to induce excessive pressure concentration. A metal band that is much wider will be difficult to shape and will probably not apply uniform pressure. The shell or band should not press on the fibular nerve. Either the component should terminate below the head of the fibula or the material should be shaped to provide a slight concavity at the bony prominence.

Most AFOs are prescribed to compensate for paralysis of the dorsiflexors. If the orthosis is intended to permit some plantar flexion or dorsiflexion, then the team should check to see that the ankle control allows the requisite motion. A metal ankle joint should be set at the level of the distal tip of the medial malleolus, the approximate site of the anatomic ankle axis. Medial and lateral joints should lie on the same axis, so that the orthosis may move smoothly. Markedly displaced ankle joints cause the calf band to slide up and down on the leg, particularly if the orthosis allows dorsiflexion.

Vertical components of the orthosis should conform to the contour of the leg without exerting undue pressure and yet not be bulky. A posterior upright should lie on the posterior midline of the leg.

If the orthosis has a patellar tendon-bearing brim, it should fit snugly without pressing uncomfortably on the skin. To test the adequacy of the brim, have the patient stand with weight equally distributed on both feet and attempt to slip a piece of paper under the shoe heel on the braced side. Effective proximal loading will allow the paper to slide under the heel.

Uprights should lie on the medial and lateral midline of the leg and thigh. Uprights that are too far posterior reduce the effectiveness of the forces applied by the calf and thigh bands. Upright placement that is too far anterior causes the calf and thigh bands to be excessively deep.

Knee-Ankle-Foot, Hip-Knee-Ankle-Foot, and Trunk-Hip-Knee-Ankle-Foot Orthoses Inspection

In addition to examining the shoe and distal components of the orthosis, the clinic team should inspect proximal elements of the KAFO and higher orthoses:

- Medial upright terminates below the perineum
- Lateral upright terminates below the greater trochanter
- Knee and hip orthotic joints coincide with anatomical counterparts
- Distal thigh band and calf shell or band are equidistant
- Ischial bearing brim is comfortable
- Trunk components are comfortable

The medial and lateral uprights contribute to control of the knee and thigh. Excessively high uprights are uncomfortable; uprights that are too low reduce the leverage that is needed for control and thus impose high forces at the proximal ends of the uprights. The orthotic knee joint should lie alongside the lateral femoral epicondyle. Although the anatomical knee has an instant center of rotation that changes as the knee is flexed, the zone of rotation is located within the epicondyle. A displaced orthotic joint may interfere with sitting comfort. The orthotic hip joint should be anterior and superior to the greater trochanter in order to coincide with the anatomic hip; otherwise, the patient may experience discomfort when sitting. Sitting comfort is also influenced by the placement of the distal thigh and calf bands. The distal margin of the distal thigh band should be equidistant from the proximal edge of the calf shell or band; otherwise, soft tissue may be compressed between the band edges, especially if the patient is obese.

An orthosis intended to limit weight-bearing through the limb must have a comfortable ischial seat with adequate room for the ischial tuberosity and sufficient relief for the adductor longus tendon. With an HKAFO or THKAFO, the pelvic band should lie flat on the torso, terminating inferiorly at the most posterior portion of the buttocks. If the band is too low, the orthosis may shift when the wearer sits. If the band is too high, the orthosis may be uncomfortable. Lateral uprights in the trunk portion of a THKAFO should lie on the lateral midline of the torso to facilitate donning and provide requisite control.

DYNAMIC EVALUATION

Assuming the orthosis fits well, the team should proceed to the dynamic phase of evaluation during which the patient walks with the orthosis. If the person is not yet able to walk, then the dynamic portion of initial evaluation will have to be postponed. If the individual can walk without the orthosis, then gait should be compared with and without the device.

One should observe the patient walking along a walkway that permits at least five strides, approximately 8 meters[1] (Table 6-1). The most efficient way of performing observational gait analysis is to focus attention only on the foot and ankle as the patient walks for several passes along the walkway. Next, observe only the action of the knee, then the hip, and finally the torso and upper limbs. Watch for movements during early stance, late stance, and swing phase, comparing the person's performance with normal gait kinematics. Observational gait analysis

TABLE 6-1

Checklist for Observing Gait

Sagittal plane deviations: Observe from the side of the patient

- Foot slap
- Toe contact
- Flat foot contact
- Excessive knee flexion
- Hyperextended knee
- Anterior trunk bending
- Posterior trunk bending
- Inadequate transition
- Toe drag
- Steppage

Frontal and transverse plane deviations: Observe from the rear of the patient

- Lateral trunk bending to affected side
- Lateral trunk bending to unaffected side
- Wide walking base
- Excessively narrow walking base
- Circumduction
- Hip hiking
- Vaulting
- Knee adduction
- Knee abduction
- Excessive medial (lateral) foot contact

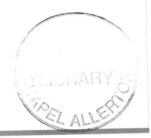

has moderate inter-rater reliability, with the greatest concurrence occurring in ratings of sagittal motions of the knee and hip.[2]

Gait analysis should be related to the purpose for which the orthosis was prescribed. For example, if the patient exhibits foot drag during swing phase without an orthosis, then the orthosis should correct this problem either by assisting dorsiflexion or preventing plantar flexion. Persistence of foot drag indicates that the orthosis has faulty alignment or a mechanical problem that needs modification. Similarly, if the patient has knee instability during early stance without an orthosis, then the orthosis should restrict knee motion. A mechanical knee lock that does not engage would expose the patient to the risk of falling because of inadvertent knee flexion.

A second consideration in dynamic evaluation is recognizing gait disorders that can be attributed to the orthosis. Some disorders must be accepted; for example, a KAFO with a knee lock will impose a stiff-legged gait, which is most conspicuous during swing phase. Patient management is thus compromised in favor of stability during stance at the expense of knee immobility during the swing phase. The gait deviation can be lessened somewhat by the addition of a 1 cm heel and sole lift on the contralateral shoe, assuming a unilateral KAFO. Another group of gait disorders caused by orthoses are those that result from faulty orthotic fit. For example, a wide walking base may be caused by excessive height of the medial upright of a KAFO. These problems demand immediate correction so that the patient does not develop bad habits.[3]

In addition to visual observation of gait, one should also listen to the patient as the individual walks. Noise may emanate from an orthosis that is malaligned or that has loose parts. Both situations may indicate premature failure of the orthosis and, in the case of malalignment, skin abrasion.

Gait Disorders During Early Stance

1. Foot slap: forefoot slaps the ground quickly and noisily
   a. Anatomical factor: weak dorsiflexors
   b. Orthotic factors: inadequate dorsiflexion assist; inadequate plantar flexion stop
2. Toe contact: initial floor contact is with the forefoot; tiptoe posture may or may not be maintained throughout the stance phase
   a. Anatomical factors: short leg, pes equinus, extensor spasticity, weak dorsiflexors, heel pain, knee and/or hip flexion contracture
   b. Orthotic factors: inadequate heel lift, inadequate dorsiflexion assist, inadequate plantar flexion stop, inadequate relief for heel pain
3. Flat foot contact: entire foot contacts the floor at initial floor contact
   a. Anatomical factor: poor balance
   b. Orthotic factors: inadequate traction from shoe sole; patient requires a walking aid, such as a cane; inadequate dorsiflexion assist; inadequate plantar flexion stop
4. Excessive medial (lateral) foot contact: medial (lateral) border of the foot contacts the floor at initial floor contact; also hyperpronation (hypersupination)
   a. Anatomical factors: weak invertors (evertors), pes valgus (varus), genu valgum (varum)
   b. Orthotic factor: transverse plane malalignment
5. Excessive knee flexion: knee collapses when the foot contacts the floor
   a. Anatomical factors: weak knee extensors, short contralateral leg, knee pain, knee and/or hip flexion contracture, flexor synergy, pes calcaneus, weak plantar flexors
   b. Orthotic factors: inadequate knee lock, inadequate dorsiflexion stop, inadequate plantar flexion stop, inadequate contralateral heel lift, requires AFO with anterior band and solid ankle, requires resilient or beveled heel
6. Hyperextended knee: patient with genu recurvatum exhibits hyperextension as weight is transferred to leg
   a. Anatomical factors: weak knee extensors; lax knee ligaments, especially collateral and anterior cruciate ligaments; extensor spasticity; pes equinus; short contralateral leg; contralateral knee and/or hip flexion contracture
   b. Orthotic factors: genu recurvatum inadequately controlled by plantar flexion stop, excessively concave calf band, pes equinus uncompensated by a contralateral shoe lift, inadequate knee lock
7. Anterior trunk bending: patient leans forward as weight is transferred to the stance leg
   a. Anatomical factors: weak knee extensors, hip flexion contracture, knee flexion contracture
   b. Orthotic factors: inadequate knee lock, requires AFO-SA with anterior band, requires resilient or beveled heel
8. Posterior trunk bending: patient leans backward as weight is transferred to the stance leg
   a. Anatomical factors: weak hip extensors, knee ankylosis
   b. Orthotic factors: inadequate hip lock, inadequate knee lock
9. Lateral trunk bending: patient leans toward the affected stance leg as weight is transferred to it. Also note whether the patient bends the trunk toward the unaffected side. Pelvis may drop or retract in response to the same factors listed here.
   a. Anatomical factors: weak hip abductors, abduction contracture, dislocated hip, hip pain, poor balance, short ipsilateral leg, amputation
   b. Orthotic factors: excessive height of the medial upright of the KAFO; excessive abduction of the hip joint of the HKAFO; insufficient heel lift; patient requires a walking aid, such as a cane
10. Abnormal walking base: heel centers are more than 10 cm apart. Also note whether the walking base is excessively narrow, less than 5 cm
    a. Anatomical factors: abduction contracture, adduction spasticity, poor balance, short contralateral leg
    b. Orthotic factors: excessive height of the medial upright of the KAFO; excessive abduction of the hip joint of the HKAFO; insufficient heel lift; patient requires a walking aid, such as a cane

Gait Disorders During Mid- and Late Stance

1. Inadequate transition: delayed transfer of weight over the forefoot
   a. Anatomical factors: weak plantar flexors, Achilles' tendon sprain or rupture, pes calcaneus, forefoot pain
   b. Orthotic factors: inadequate plantar flexion stop, inadequate dorsiflexion stop, patient requires a rocker bar on the shoe sole
2. Knee adduction (abduction): knee increases valgus or varus alignment
   a. Anatomical factors: ligamentous laxity, weak medial (lateral) quadriceps and/or hamstrings, arthritic changes
   b. Orthotic factors: malalignment of uprights of KAFO, need for medial (lateral) calf shell extension or five-strap knee pad

Gait Disorders During Swing Phase

1. Toe drag: toes contact the floor
   a. Anatomical factors: weak dorsiflexors, extensor spasticity, pes equinus, weak hip flexors, knee and/or ankle ankylosis
   b. Orthotic factors: inadequate dorsiflexion assist, inadequate plantar flexion stop
2. Steppage: hip flexion is exaggerated in excursion and/or duration
   a. Anatomical factors: weak dorsiflexors, pes equinus, ankle ankylosis

   b. Orthotic factors: inadequate dorsiflexion assist, inadequate plantar flexion stop
3. Circumduction: leg swings outward in a semi circular arc
   a. Anatomical factors: weak dorsiflexors, weak hip flexors, extensor spasticity, pes equinus, knee and/or ankle ankylosis, short contralateral leg, inadequate weight shift, contralateral knee and/or hip flexion con tracture
   b. Orthotic factors: knee lock, inadequate dorsiflexion assist, inadequate plantar flex ion stop
4. Hip hiking: pelvis elevates to enable the limb to swing forward
5. Vaulting: exaggerated plantar flexion of the contralateral leg enables the ipsilateral limb to swing forward (Note: Same anatomical and orthotic factors as for hip hiking and circum-duction)

REFERENCES

1. Rose JR, Gamble JG, eds. *Human Walking*. 2nd ed. Baltimore, Md: Williams & Wilkins; 1994.
2. Krebs DE, Edelstein JE, Fishman S. Reliability of observational kinematic gait analysis. *Phys Ther.* 1985;65:1027-1033.
3. Edelstein JE. Prosthetic and orthotic gait. In: Smidt GL, ed. *Gait in Rehabilitation*. New York, NY: Churchill Livingstone; 1990.

Chapter 7

Trunk and Cervical Orthoses

I, that am rudely stamp'd, and want love's majesty
To strut before a wanton ambling nymph;
I, that am curtail'd of this fair proportion
Cheated of feature by dissembling nature,
Deform'd, unfinish'd, sent before my time
Into this breathing world scarce half made up.
William Shakespeare, King Richard III

Orthoses for the neck and trunk are often prescribed to reduce pain and minimize deformity. They affect the body primarily by resisting motion or protecting the body part, rather than assisting motion or transferring force, as is the case with orthoses for the limbs.

TRUNK ORTHOSES

The clinical utility of trunk orthoses is controversial because well-controlled studies are difficult to conduct. Anecdotal evidence, however, suggests that some patients experience pain reduction and thus achieve greater function while wearing an orthosis. Trunk musculature may relax when the individual uses an orthosis. In addition, limiting motion through the pain-free excursion helps the patient resume customary activity. For the short-term, the therapeutic effect is desirable; however, if the trunk orthosis is worn for an extended period, the patient will develop disuse atrophy and weakness. The psychosocial effects of trunk orthoses cannot be ignored: the orthosis is a visible indicator of disability.

Although the intended purpose may be to influence the position or the motion of the vertebral column, the designation "spinal orthosis" is misleading. The orthosis is worn over soft tissue and usually over the pelvis or thorax, or both bony structures. Consequently, "trunk orthosis" is a more accurate term. Even when the therapeutic intention is to affect the spine, the forces that an orthosis apply are dissipated by the skin and underlying tissues. Skin tolerance is a major factor limiting the snugness with which an orthosis can be worn.

As noted in Chapter 1, "orthosis" refers to any appliance worn on the body for therapeutic purposes. Nevertheless, the most commonly used trunk orthoses are often called "corsets" or "belts." These terms connote orthoses that lack rigid horizontal structures; often, the corset or belt does have vertical reinforcements.

Orthoses for the trunk are usually mass-produced. Patients with marked trunk deformity or unusual size may require custom-made appliances.

Most orthoses worn on the trunk compress the abdomen, thereby increasing intra-abdominal pressure. Some orthoses also restrict motion in one or

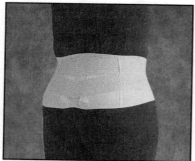

Figure 7-1. Sacroiliac corset—posterior view (reprinted with permission of CAMP Healthcare).

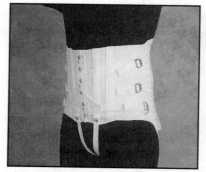

Figure 7-2. Lumbosacral corset—anterior view (reproduced with permission of CAMP Healthcare).

more planes. Generic names used to designate specific orthoses reflect the biomechanical effect as well as the region of the trunk covered by the orthosis, namely sacroiliac, lumbosacral, and thoracolumbosacral.

Sacroiliac Orthoses

Sacroiliac orthoses are corsets (Figure 7-1). Because of their relatively narrow width, they are often called belts. They encircle the lower portion of the torso. The superior termination is ordinarily just below the level of the iliac crests, and the bottom edge is at the level of the inguinal ligaments. Belts for men are usually made with groin straps to prevent the appliance from displacing upward. For women, the belt may have garters intended to be secured to stockings so that the orthosis keeps in place. Belts are made of lightweight canvas or similar fabric and may have short vertical reinforcing stays to prevent the belt from forming horizontal creases. Most belts are mass-produced in a large range of sizes to fit adults having many different body configurations.

Belts are usually prescribed to reduce sacroiliac diastasis or pubic symphysis separation, such as occasionally occurs in pregnancy. Sacroiliac orthoses may be issued on a prophylactic basis to workers who engage in heavy lifting, such as delivery agents and nursing home attendants. In addition to resisting stresses on the symphysis and posterior joints, the belt may also reduce tension in the spinal extensor musculature in the lumbosacral region.[1] Of course, any therapeutic benefit is negated if the wearer fails to secure the belt snugly.

Lumbosacral Orthoses

Corsets

Corsets are probably the most frequently worn trunk orthoses. A lumbosacral corset (Figure 7-2) encircles the torso from the level of the xiphoid process to the pubic symphysis. Posteriorly, the corset extends from a point just below the inferior angles of the scapulae to the apices of the buttocks. The corset may have a rigid plastic plate inserted into a posterior pocket. The plate is molded on the patient and acts primarily to restrict trunk hyperextension.[2] A corset compresses the abdomen, increasing intracavitary pressure, thereby reducing stress on the spinal extensors. The individual who experiences muscle spasms in the lower back may find pain relief as the postural demand on the spinal musculature lessens.[3,4] Orthoses can also improve the wearer's awareness of proprioception.[5] Corsets restrict pelvic motion in the sagittal and transverse planes minimally but do limit frontal plane motion to a moderate extent.[6]

Lumbosacral Flexion Extension Control Orthosis

The lumbosacral flexion extension control orthosis (LS FEO) (Figure 7-3) covers the same portion of the trunk as does the lumbosacral corset. The orthosis was originally called a chairback brace. It includes rigid or semirigid horizontal and vertical components. The thoracic band should be positioned horizontally on the back just below the scapulae. The

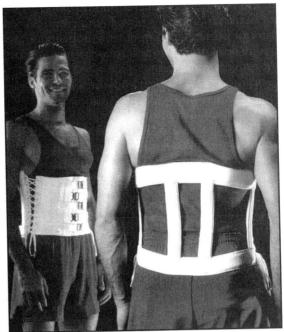

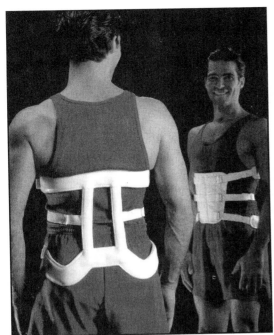

Figure 7-3. Lumbosacral flexion extension control orthosis (reproduced with permission of Becker Orthopedic).

Figure 7-4. Lumbosacral flexion extension lateral control orthosis (reproduced with permission of Becker Orthopedic).

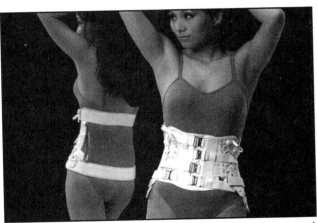

Figure 7-5. Lumbosacral extension lateral control orthosis.

pelvic band should be curved to cover the apex of each buttock and should lie flat over the sacrum. The bands are connected by a pair of posterior uprights placed on either side of the vertebral spinous processes. A sturdy fabric abdominal front attached to the posterior uprights completes the orthosis.

The orthosis restricts trunk flexion by a three-point force system consisting of posteriorly directed forces from the top and bottom of the abdominal front and an anteriorly directed force from the center of the posterior uprights. Hyperextension is restricted by anteriorly directed forces from the thoracic and

pelvic bands and a posteriorly directed force from the midsection of the abdominal front.[7]

Lumbosacral Flexion Extension Lateral Control Orthosis

The lumbosacral flexion extension lateral control orthosis (LS FELO) (Figure 7-4) resembles the LS FEO with the addition of a lateral upright on each side. The LS FELO was formerly known as a Knight spinal brace.

The same pressure systems restrict trunk flexion and hyperextension in both the LS FEO and the LS FELO. The latter orthosis also restricts lateral flexion by means of the lateral uprights. Trunk bending to the right is limited by a three-point system consisting of leftward forces from the top and bottom of the right lateral upright and a rightward force from the middle of the left lateral upright.[8]

Lumbosacral Extension Lateral Control Orthosis

The lumbosacral extension lateral control orthosis (LS ELO) (Figure 7-5), also called a Williams brace, consists of a pelvic band, thoracic band, and lateral uprights. The lateral uprights are attached by pivots to the thoracic band. Instead of posterior uprights, the orthosis has a pair of oblique uprights, each of which extends from the pelvic band to the upper third of a lateral upright. In front is an elastic abdominal front.

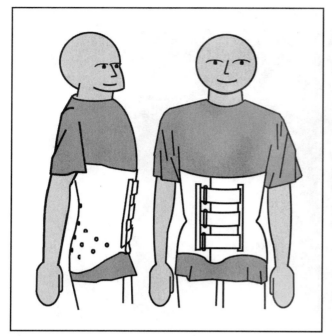

Figure 7-6. Lumbosacral flexion extension lateral rotary control orthosis.

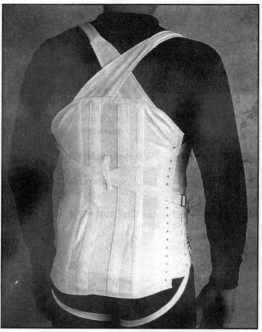

Figure 7-7. Thoracolumbosacral corset (reproduced with permission of CAMP Healthcare).

The LS ELO restricts trunk hyperextension by anteriorly directed force from the thoracic and pelvic bands and a posteriorly directed force from the midsection of the abdominal front. Lacking posterior uprights, the LS ELO does not limit trunk flexion appreciably. Lateral uprights restrict sideward bending. The orthosis was designed to discourage a hyperlordotic posture and is intended to be used with trunk flexion exercises.

Lumbosacral Flexion Extension Lateral Rotary Control Orthosis

Restriction of all motions of the lower trunk can be achieved by a semirigid plastic jacket called a lumbosacral flexion extension lateral rotary control orthosis (LS FELRO) (Figure 7-6). Although the lumbar vertebrae do not permit much motion in the transverse plane, this orthosis restricts whatever rotary motion may exist.[3,4,9-12]

Thoracolumbosacral Orthoses

Most thoracolumbosacral (TLS) orthoses have axillary straps extending from a fabric or a rigid posterior section, passing through the axillae to the front of the chest, and continuing back to terminate posteriorly.

Thoracolumbosacral Corsets

Thoracolumbosacral corsets (Figure 7-7) have a posterior section extending upward, which serves as the attachment point for the axillary straps. The inferior trimline is the same as for the lumbosacral corset and may include either groin straps or garters. In front, the male version of the TLS corset terminates at about the same point as does the LS corset. The TLS corset for women includes a brassiere. The TLS corset increases intra-abdominal pressure and provides minimal restriction against trunk flexion and hyperextension.

Thoracolumbosacral Flexion Extension Control Orthosis

The thoracolumbosacral flexion extension control orthosis (TLS FEO) (Figure 7-8), also known as the Taylor brace, includes a pelvic band, posterior uprights that terminate above the scapular spines, an abdominal front secured to the posterior uprights, and axillary straps. An interscapular band secured to the posterior uprights lies horizontally above the scapular spines.

The orthosis limits trunk flexion by means of posteriorly directed forces from the axillary straps and the lower border of the abdominal front and an anteriorly directed force from the center of the posterior uprights. Hyperextension is restricted by anteriorly directed forces from the pelvic and interscapular bands and a posteriorly directed force from the midsection of the abdominal front.

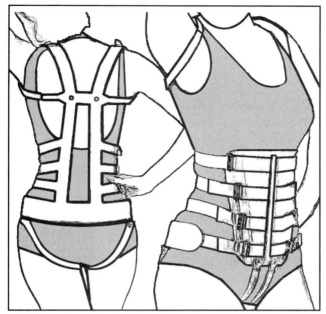

Figure 7-8. Thoracolumbosacral flexion extension control orthosis.

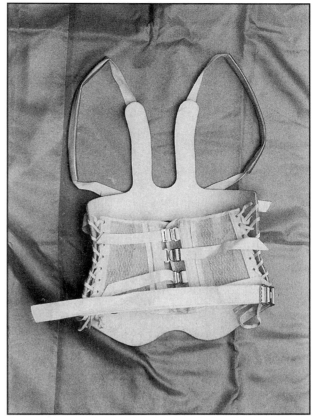

Figure 7-9a. Thoracolumbosacral flexion extension lateral control orthosis—anterior aspect.

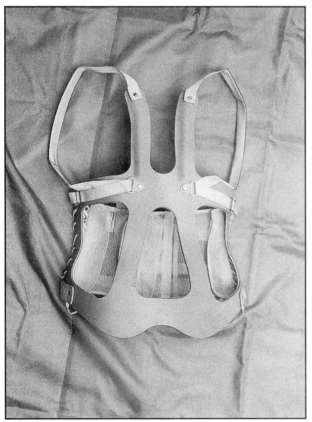

Figure 7-9b. Thoracolumbosacral flexion extension lateral control orthosis—posterior aspect.

Thoracolumbosacral Flexion Extension Lateral Control Orthosis

A more restrictive orthosis is the thoracolumbosacral flexion extension lateral control orthosis (TLS FELO) (Figures 7-9a and 7-9b), also called the Knight-Taylor brace. Similar to the TLS FEO, the TLS FELO has a thoracic band, rather than the interscapular band, and lateral uprights.

The TLS FELO restricts trunk flexion with posteriorly directed forces from the axillary straps and the lower border of the abdominal front and an anteriorly directed force from the center of the posterior uprights. Hyperextension is restricted by anteriorly directed force from the pelvic and thoracic bands and a posteriorly directed force from the midsection of the abdominal front. Lateral uprights minimize lateral flexion.

Thoracolumbosacral Flexion Control Orthosis

A trunk orthosis that does not cover the abdomen is the thoracolumbosacral flexion control orthosis (TLS FO) (Figures 7-10a and 7-10b). This mass-produced appliance is made in two designs, both of

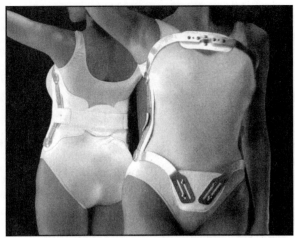

Figure 7-10a. Thoracolumbosacral flexion control orthosis—lateral uprights design (reproduced with permission of Becker Orthopedic).

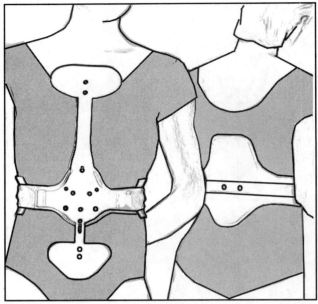

Figure 7-10b. Thoracolumbosacral flexion control orthosis—cruciform design (reproduced with permission of Becker Orthopedic).

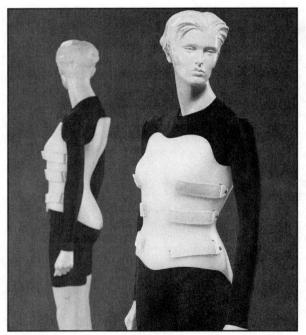

Figure 7-11. Thoracolumbosacral flexion extension lateral rotary control orthosis (reproduced with permission of Spinal Technology, Inc.).

which apply the same three-point force system to restrict forward bending. One version includes sternal and suprapubic plates in front and a dorsolumbar plate posteriorly. The plates are joined by a rigid frame designed to lie slightly away from the torso. Altering plate position is facilitated by numerous screw holes on the plates and frame. Another version is cruciform and features sternal and suprapubic plates connected by an anterior vertical upright. A

cross piece on the upright has straps that encircle the waist; the straps anchor a dorsolumbar plate. This design is somewhat easier for the patient to don.

The TLS FO is intended primarily for adults with thoracic vertebral body fracture. It significantly reduces segmental as well as gross spinal movement.[13] It is also prescribed for patients with thoracic spinal cord injury in which trunk stabilization with maximum skin exposure is sought.

Thoracolumbosacral Flexion Extension Lateral Rotary Control Orthosis

The most restrictive TLS orthosis is the thoracolumbosacral flexion extension lateral rotary control orthosis (TLS FELRO) (Figure 7-11). The most common version is a plastic jacket that encircles the torso from the groin to the upper chest. The jacket may be custom-made, usually from polyethylene molded over a plaster model of the patient's trunk. Alternatively, the patient may be fitted with a mass-produced jacket, which is adjusted on an individual basis. One type of TLS FELRO has a posterior inflatable pad intended to enable the patient to adjust the snugness and pressure applied by the orthosis.

Another version of TLS FELRO is known colloquially as the cowhorn brace. It is essentially a TLS FELO with anterior extensions of the thoracic band, which terminate in subclavicular pads. It restricts thoracic rotation to the right by posteriorly directed force from the right subclavicular pad and anteriorly

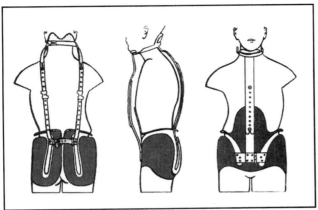

Figure 7-12. Foundation of the Milwaukee orthosis with thoracic pads to be added on an individual basis.

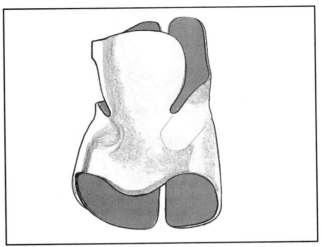

Figure 7-13. Boston orthosis (reproduced with permission of Boston Brace International, Inc.).

directed force to the left side of the thoracic band. This force couple is complemented by a second one consisting of posteriorly directed force from the left lower portion of the abdominal front and anteriorly directed force from the pelvic band on the right side.

TRUNK ORTHOSIS EVALUATION

- Orthosis is comfortable
- Pelvic band lies between the posterior superior iliac spines and posterior margin of the buttocks
- Thoracic band lies below the scapulae
- Thoracic band lies horizontal
- Posterior uprights do not contact the spinous processes
- Each lateral upright lies on the lateral midline of the torso
- Abdominal front extends from the xiphoid process to the pubic symphysis
- Suprapubic plate lies between the anterior superior iliac spines and the pubic symphysis
- Sternal plate lies between the jugular notch and the sternal angle

SCOLIOSIS AND KYPHOSIS ORTHOSES

A special group of TLS orthoses is designed for children and adolescents who have scoliosis or kyphosis. Unlike the preceding appliances, which are prescribed for adults to wear during the day for a few weeks, scoliosis orthoses are customarily intended to be worn until the patient reaches spinal maturity. They are meant to be worn 16 to 23 hours daily. They are most effective with patients who have

lateral curves between 20 and 45 degrees with the apex no higher than the sixth thoracic vertebra.

The Milwaukee orthosis (Figure 7-12) is the oldest scoliosis orthosis in contemporary use in the United States. Invented by Richard Bidwell, CO, and Walter Blount, MD, in Milwaukee, Wis., in the 1940s, it is still frequently prescribed for youngsters with juvenile or adolescent scoliosis. This custom-made orthosis consists of a pelvic girdle and a neck ring joined in front with a single metal upright and in back by a pair of uprights. Because the neck ring may include an occipital plate, the orthosis is sometimes called a cervicothoracolumbosacral orthosis (CTLSO). The newest model of neck ring lies on the upper chest, making it easy to conceal under clothing and eliminating the risk of mandibular pressure. These were problems associated with earlier designs of the Milwaukee orthosis. The superstructure serves as the attachment point for various pads, which provide passive control of the spinal curvature. The patient may also achieve active control by moving away from the pads at frequent intervals during the day. Most Milwaukee orthoses include an "L"-shaped thoracic pad placed over the apex of the thoracic curve. A lumbar pad is another common component.

Patients with adolescent kyphosis are sometimes fitted with a Milwaukee orthosis that has a kyphosis pad placed on each posterior upright at the apex of the curve.

A newer alternate to the Milwaukee orthosis is the Boston orthosis (Figure 7-13), invented at Children's Hospital, Boston, Mass., by William Hall, CO.[14] This TLS O is sometimes designated as "low profile" because it does not have a neck ring. It is thus less

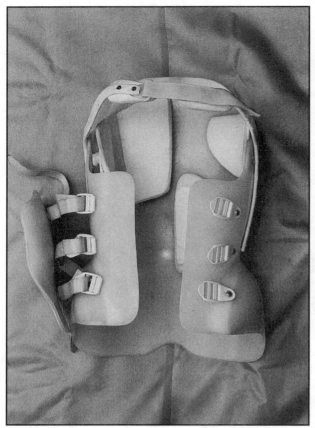

Figure 7-14. New York Orthopaedic Hospital orthosis. This model is missing the thoracic pads.

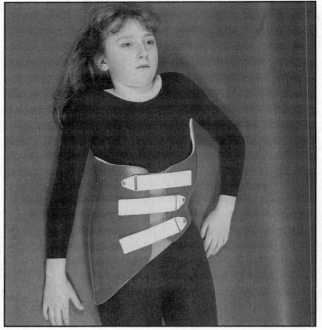

Figure 7-15. Providence orthosis on supine child (reproduced with permission of Spinal Technology, Inc.).

conspicuous than the Milwaukee orthosis, a practical consideration for adolescent patients. It differs from the Milwaukee orthosis in several other respects. First, the Boston orthosis is made from a plastic module that is manufactured in a large range of sizes. Second, pressure pads are secured inside the module to apply controlling forces to the trunk. A variation of the Boston orthosis is beneficial for patients who have spondylolysis and spondylolisthesis.[15]

Other low-profile scoliosis orthoses include the Wilmington and the New York Orthopaedic Hospital orthoses. The Wilmington orthosis was invented at DuPont Children's Hospital, Wilmington, Del. The New York Orthopaedic Hospital orthosis (Figure 7-14) was designed at Columbia Medical Center in New York City. Both orthoses feature an anterior opening that facilitates donning. The Wilmington orthosis is a custom-made plastic jacket molded over a plaster model of the torso, which is taken while the patient is held in the position of maximum passive correction. The New York Orthopaedic Hospital orthosis is also custom-made; it has corrective pads secured on the interior of the plastic jacket.

Regardless of orthosis, its efficacy is strongly influenced by how tightly the orthosis is fastened and the location and design of its pressure pads.[16]

The preceding orthoses are intended for day-and-night wear with brief respites for bathing and exercise. More recently, several orthoses have been designed for use only when the patient is recumbent. The two most prominent are the Charleston bending brace and the Providence Scoliosis System (Figure 7-15). The Charleston orthosis positions the trunk in overcorrection. The Providence orthosis is molded with a low inferior trimline on the contralateral side and a high superior trimline on the ipsilateral side of the apex of the curve. Limited clinical experience suggests that these orthoses produce results comparable to that achieved with the Milwaukee orthosis and similar appliances.[17-20]

SCOLIOSIS AND KYPHOSIS ORTHOSIS EVALUATION

- Pelvic girdle terminates above the pubic symphysis and the greater trochanter
- Pelvic girdle does not exert excessive pressure over the iliac crests
- Pelvic girdle compresses the abdomen

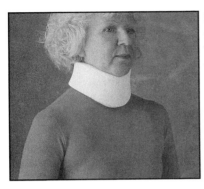

Figure 7-16. Soft collar (reproduced with permission of CAMP Healthcare).

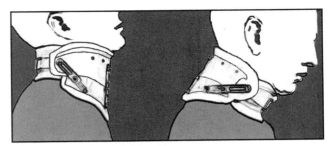

Figure 7-17. Semirigid collar.

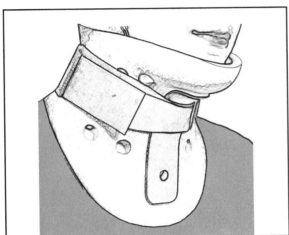

Figure 7-18. Philadelphia collar.

- Occipital pads lie just below the occipital tuberosities
- Lumbar, thoracic, and kyphosis pads apply firm pressure to the apices of the curvatures
- Uprights allow for chest expansion during respiration

CERVICAL ORTHOSES

Orthoses for the neck can be classified as collars, post devices, or maximum immobilizing orthoses. Cervical appliances differ in appearance and in the extent to which they restrict neck motion. They are almost always mass-produced.

Collars

Flexible or semirigid orthoses, sometimes termed soft collars (Figure 7-16), are made of solid material and wrap around the neck. Often, a collar is a broad strip of foam rubber, foam plastic, or felt encased in cotton stockinette and secured with hook-and-pile tape. Polyethylene sheeting is occasionally used for semirigid collars (Figure 7-17). Some collars have

vertical stays that slightly restrict motion. Even with reinforcement, collars are the least restrictive of any cervical orthosis.[21,22] They remind the wearer to avoid abrupt movement. They also retain heat, which may reduce the incidence and severity of muscle spasm.

One version of collar is known as the Philadelphia collar (Figure 7-18). It was developed in 1971 by Anthony Calabrese, an orthotist in Philadelphia, Pa. Manufactured of polyethylene foam with an anterior vertical reinforcement, the collar extends from the chin to the manubrium in front and from the occipital tuberosities to the region above the scapular spines in back. Some designs have a hole in front through which a tracheotomy tube may be inserted. The Philadelphia collar is more restrictive than the ordinary collar, particularly when the wearer attempts to flex the neck. A snugly fitted version of the Philadelphia collar can be used to control hypertrophic scarring in patients with burn wounds on the neck.

Post Orthoses

Cervical orthoses that include rigid vertical posts are more restrictive and cooler than collars. Such orthoses have superior portions that contact the chin and occiput, and inferior portions that lie on the chest and upper back. The front and back components of the superior portion are buckled. Similarly, the front and back components of the inferior portion are buckled to enable donning and adjustment, and have shoulder straps to stabilize the orthosis. Posts extend between the superior and inferior portions. In most instances, the posts are adjustable so that the posture of the head may be controlled.

The two-post orthosis (Figure 7-19) has anterior and posterior midline posts. This orthosis restricts neck flexion and extension but is much less effective in limiting cervical rotation or lateral flexion.

A three-post orthosis (Figure 7-20) is also known as the sternal-occipital-mandibular immobilizer (SOMI). It has a midline anterior post terminating in a mandibular plate. The two other posts are curved

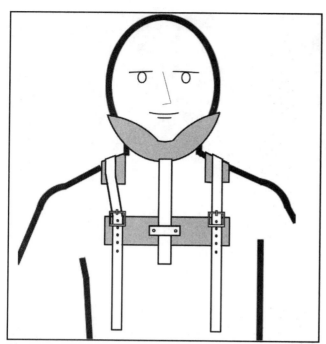

Figure 7-19. Two-post orthosis.

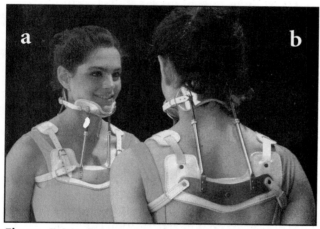

Figure 7-21. Four-post orthosis: a. Anterior aspect. b. Posterior aspect.

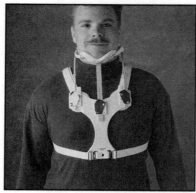

Figure 7-20. Three-post orthosis—sterno-occipital-mandibular immobilizer (reproduced with permission of CAMP Healthcare).

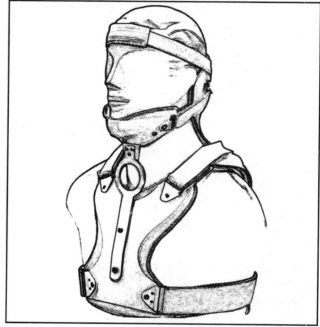

Figure 7-22. Minerva orthosis.

and extend from a chest plate to each side of the occipital plate. The orthosis is designed to be applied to the supine patient without turning the neck. The SOMI is particularly effective in limiting neck flexion. A variation of the SOMI substitutes a forehead band for the mandibular plate.

The four-post orthosis (Figure 7-21) has anterior and posterior posts set on either side of the mandibular and occipital plates. Consequently, it restricts neck rotation and lateral flexion in addition to flexion and extension.[23-25]

Maximum Immobilizing Orthoses

Patients with cervical fracture—with or without spinal cord injury—are often fitted with orthoses that limit neck motion to a marked extent. These orthoses are prescribed to prevent aggravation of the patient's neuromusculoskeletal condition. Such devices may be noninvasive, worn on the outside of the head and chest; or invasive, having pins inserted into the cranial vault.[26]

Noninvasive orthoses include the Minerva and cuirass designs. The Minerva orthosis (Figure 7-22) may be custom-made or mass-produced. It has a semirigid anterior section extending from the mid-chest to the chin and a semirigid posterior section that extends from the mid-dorsum to the parietal area of the skull. The posterior section has a padded

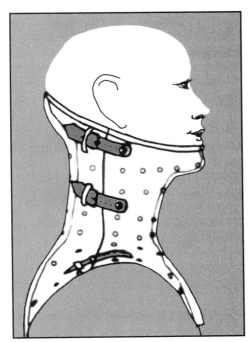

Figure 7-23. Cuirass orthosis.

band that extends forward to encircle the forehead.[27] The name refers to the mythological Roman goddess Minerva, favorite daughter of Zeus. She is described as a fierce combatant who radiated thunderbolts from her forehead. She is also the embodiment of wisdom. The forehead band thus alludes both to her cerebral lightning and intelligence.

The cuirass orthosis (Figure 7-23) is usually custom-made of semirigid plastic. The anterior chest section is similar to that of the Minerva orthosis. The posterior section terminates superiorly at the occipitoparietal margin of the skull. The name "cuirass" suggests the leather-lined medieval armor that was worn to surround and protect the head and neck. The cuirass orthosis is sometimes used to prevent neck contracture subsequent to burns or torticollis.

The most frequently prescribed orthosis for maximum immobilization is the halo (Figure 7-24), an invasive type of post appliance. It consists of a rigid ring joined by four posts to anterior and posterior chest plates. An orthopedist secures the ring by means of four screws placed in holes drilled through the scalp, subcutaneous tissue, epicranial aponeurosis, and pericranial outer table of compact bone. Because four pins stabilize the ring, it is not necessary that the pins penetrate far into the skull. The orthotist adjusts the height of the posts to achieve the desired neck posture. The chest plates are usually lined with sheepskin to minimize pressure concentration. The name of the orthosis refers to the ring

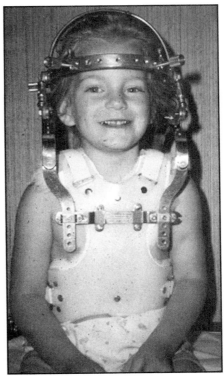

Figure 7-24. Halo orthosis (reproduced with permission of Fillauer, Inc.).

that resembles a halo. This orthosis offers maximum immobilization of neck motion in all directions. Because it impairs the wearer's balance control, it may increase the risk of falling.[28]

CERVICAL ORTHOSIS EVALUATION

- Head is in the appropriate position
- Sternal plate lies between the jugular notch and the sternal angle
- Occipital pads lie just below the occipital tuberosities
- Mandibular plate applies uniform pressure to the chin
- Thoracic plate does not contact the scapular spines

GUIDELINES FOR PRESCRIPTION

The following are biomechanical guidelines for prescribing trunk and cervical orthoses:

1. To reduce stress on trunk extensors by compressing the abdomen, the following orthoses include an abdominal front. Selection depends

on the size of abdominal front deemed appropriate for the patient and the amount, if any, of additional motion restriction that may be beneficial.
a. Sacroiliac corset
b. Lumbosacral corset
c. Lumbosacral flexion extension control orthosis
d. Lumbosacral flexion extension lateral control orthosis
e. Lumbosacral extension lateral control orthosis
f. Lumbosacral flexion extension lateral rotary control orthosis
g. Thoracolumbosacral corset
h. Thoracolumbosacral flexion extension control orthosis
i. Thoracolumbosacral flexion extension lateral control orthosis
j. Thoracolumbosacral flexion extension lateral rotary control orthosis
2. To restrict trunk flexion, the following orthoses include an abdominal front or sternal and suprapubic pads and posterior uprights, or a posterior section. Selection depends on the trunk area that should be restricted and the amount, if any, of additional motion restriction that may be beneficial.
a. Lumbosacral flexion extension control orthosis
b. Lumbosacral flexion extension lateral control orthosis
c. Lumbosacral flexion extension lateral rotary control orthosis
d. Thoracolumbosacral flexion control orthosis
e. Thoracolumbosacral flexion extension control orthosis
f. Thoracolumbosacral flexion extension lateral control orthosis
g. Thoracolumbosacral flexion extension lateral rotary control orthosis
3. To restrict trunk extension, the following orthoses include an abdominal front and thoracic and pelvic bands. Selection depends on the trunk area that should be restricted and the amount of additional motion restriction that may be beneficial.
a. Lumbosacral flexion extension control orthosis
b. Lumbosacral flexion extension lateral control orthosis
c. Lumbosacral flexion extension lateral rotary control orthosis

d. Lumbosacral extension lateral control orthosis
e. Thoracolumbosacral flexion extension control orthosis
f. Thoracolumbosacral flexion extension lateral control orthosis
g. Thoracolumbosacral flexion extension lateral rotary control orthosis
4. To restrict trunk lateral bending, the following orthoses include lateral uprights. Selection depends on the trunk area that should be restricted and the amount of additional motion restriction that may be beneficial.
a. Lumbosacral flexion extension lateral control orthosis
b. Lumbosacral extension lateral control orthosis
c. Lumbosacral flexion extension lateral rotary control orthosis
d. Thoracolumbosacral flexion extension lateral control orthosis
e. Thoracolumbosacral flexion extension lateral rotary control orthosis
5. To restrict trunk rotation, the following orthoses include rigid sections that encircle the torso. Selection depends on the trunk area that should be restricted.
a. Lumbosacral flexion extension lateral rotary control orthosis
b. Thoracolumbosacral flexion extension lateral rotary control orthosis
6. To control scoliosis and kyphosis day and night, the following orthoses include sections that stabilize the pelvis and thorax. The Milwaukee and Boston orthoses also have pads that apply corrective forces. Selection depends on the trunk area to be controlled.
a. Milwaukee orthosis
b. Boston orthosis
c. New York Orthopaedic Hospital orthosis
d. Wilmington orthosis
7. To control scoliosis and kyphosis only at night, the following orthoses place the torso in a position opposite to that of the deformity. Selection depends on the extent of trunk coverage that may be beneficial.
a. Charleston orthosis
b. Providence orthosis
8. To provide minimal limitation of neck motion, the following orthoses encircle the neck. Selection depends on the amount of limitation and the extent of neck coverage that may be beneficial.

a. Soft collar
b. Hard collar

9. To limit neck flexion, the following orthoses include anterior and posterior rigid uprights or solid structures. Selection depends on the amount of limitation, the additional motion restriction, and the amount of coverage that may be beneficial.
   a. Philadelphia collar
   b. Two-post orthosis
   c. Three-post orthosis (sterno-occipital-mandibular immobilizer)
   d. Four-post orthosis
   e. Minerva orthosis
   f. Cuirass orthosis
   g. Halo orthosis

10. To limit neck extension, the following orthoses include anterior and posterior rigid uprights or solid structures. Selection depends on the amount of limitation, the additional motion restriction, and the amount of coverage that may be beneficial.
    a. Two-post orthosis
    b. Four-post orthosis
    c. Minerva orthosis
    d. Cuirass orthosis
    e. Halo orthosis

11. To limit neck lateral flexion and rotation, the following orthoses include lateral uprights or solid sections. Selection depends on the amount of limitation, the additional motion restriction, and the amount of coverage that may be beneficial.
    a. Four-post orthosis
    b. Minerva orthosis
    c. Cuirass orthosis
    d. Halo orthosis

SUMMARY

Orthoses for the trunk are usually prescribed to reduce pain caused by muscle tension or movement through an extreme range. Although short-term pain relief is desirable, prolonged reliance on a trunk orthosis can lead to disuse atrophy, weakness, and psychological dependency. Because orthoses are worn on the outside of the body, forces that may be intended to influence the position of the vertebral column are dissipated by skin and soft tissue. Skin tolerance limits the snugness and the forces that the orthosis can apply.

Sacroiliac, lumbosacral, and thoracolumbosacral regions may be encompassed by a trunk orthosis. Corsets, sometimes called belts, are orthoses that do not have rigid horizontal components. Sacroiliac corsets are prescribed to reduce sacroiliac diastasis or pubic symphysis separation, or as a preventive measure against low back strain for workers required to lift people or heavy objects. Lumbosacral orthoses include corsets and orthoses limiting flexion and extension; flexion, extension, and lateral motion; extension and lateral motion; and flexion, extension, lateral, and rotary motion. Typically, these orthoses include pelvic and thoracic bands and a fabric abdominal front, which increases intracavitary pressure to reduce demand on trunk extensors. Most orthoses also have posterior uprights, while some also have lateral uprights. Motion control is achieved by means of a series of three-point pressure systems (eg, flexion control requires anteriorly directed force from the midportion of the posterior uprights and posteriorly directed force from the top and bottom of the abdominal front).

Thoracolumbosacral orthoses include corsets, as well as rigid orthoses limiting flexion and extension; flexion, extension, and lateral motion; flexion; and flexion, extension, lateral, and rotary motion. The TLS flexion control orthosis lacks an abdominal front and is prescribed to limit compressive forces on thoracic vertebral bodies.

Scoliosis and kyphosis orthoses include the Milwaukee orthosis, as well as those designed in Boston, New York, and Wilmington, all of which maintain the torso in a position of maximum correction and are intended to be worn 16 to 23 hours a day until the patient reaches skeletal maturity. Providence and Charleston orthoses place the trunk in a position of overcorrection and are designed for night wear when the patient is recumbent.

Cervical orthoses are appliances that limit motion of the neck to varying extents and in various direction. Collars, whether flexible or semirigid, encircle the neck and remind the wearer to avoid excessive movement. The Philadelphia collar restricts neck motion. Post orthoses provide greater motion restriction; they include two-, three-, and four-post orthoses, the last being most restrictive. Maximum immobilization of the neck is achieved with noninvasive orthoses such as the Minerva and the cuirass, and by the halo orthosis, which is secured to the skull.

THOUGHT QUESTIONS

1. Elastic trunk supports have become popular for people in express mail delivery services and for baggage handlers at airports. What is your opinion regarding these supports for such workers? How might they help prevent back

injury? Do they promote muscle atrophy? Explain your answer.

2. Would you recommend that a postmenopausal woman with a family history of osteoporosis wear a corset to prevent compression fractures of her spine? Explain your answer.

3. Many adolescent girls with idiopathic scoliosis would rather tolerate a mild spinal curvature than feel humiliated by appearing in school with an orthosis. Describe several strategies that can be used to facilitate scoliosis management with these patients.

4. Describe the pressure/force system inherent in a lumbosacral corset.

5. Describe three different patients for whom you would order a soft collar.

REFERENCES

1. Van Poppel MN, Koes BW, van der Ploeg T. Lumbar supports and education for the prevention of low back pain in industry. *JAMA*. 1998;279:1789-1794.

2. Deamer RM, Anderson RB. Improved orthotic low-back support for help with low-back pain. *Journal of Prosthetics and Orthotics*. 1997;9:38-41.

3. Lantz S, Schultz A. Lumbar spine orthosis wearing: effects on trunk muscle myoelectric activity. *Spine*. 1986;11:838-842.

4. Lantz S, Schultz A. Lumbar spine orthosis wearing: restriction of gross body motion. *Spine*. 1986;11:834-837.

5. McNair PJ, Heine PJ. Trunk proprioception: enhancement through lumbar brace. *Arch Phys Med Rehabil*. 1999;80:96-99.

6. Vogt L, Pfeifer K, Portscher M, Banzer W. Lumbar corsets: their effect on three-dimensional kinematics of the pelvis. *J Rehabil Res Dev*. 2000;37:495-499.

7. Spratt KF, Weinstein JN, Lehmann TR, Woody J, Sayre H. Efficacy of flexion and extension treatments incorporating braces for low-back pain patients with retrodisplacement, spondylolisthesis, or normal sagittal translation. *Spine*. 1993;18:1839-1849.

8. Tuong H, Dansereau J, Maurais G, Herrera R. Three-dimensional evaluation of lumbar orthosis effects on spinal behavior. *J Rehabil Res Dev*. 1998;35:34-42.

9. Bell DF, Ehrlich MG, Zaleski DJ. Brace treatment for symptomatic spondylolisthesis. *Clin Orthop*. 1989;142:538-540.

10. Fidler MW, Plasmans MT. The effect of four types of support on the segmental mobility of the lumbosacral joint. *J Bone Joint Surg [Am]*. 1983;65:943-947.

11. Sinaki M, Lutness MP, Ilstrup DM, Chu CP, Gramse RR. Lumbar spondylolisthesis: retrospective comparison and three-year follow-up of two conservative treatment programs. *Arch Phys Med Rehabil*. 1989;70:594-598.

12. Smith KM. A preliminary report on a new design of a spinal orthosis for spondylitic patients: review of the literature and initiation for future study of a new design. *Journal of Prosthetics and Orthotics*. 1998;10:45-49.

13. Van Leeuwen PJ, Bos RP, Derksen JC, de Vries J. Assessment of spinal movement reduction by thoraco-lumbar-sacral orthoses. *J Rehabil Res Dev*. 2000;37:35-403.

14. Olafsson Y, Saraste H, Soderlund V, Hoffsten M. Boston brace in the treatment of idiopathic scoliosis. *J Pediatr Orthop*. 1995;15:524-527.

15. Steiner ME, Micheli LJ. Treatment of symptomatic spondylolysis and spondylolisthesis with the modified Boston brace. *Spine*. 1985;10:937-943.

16. Wong MS, Mak AFT, Luk KDK, et al. Effectiveness and biomechanics of spinal orthoses in the treatment of adolescent idiopathic scoliosis. *Prosthet Orthot Int*. 2000;24:148-162.

17. Montgomery F, Willner S, Appelgren G. Long-term follow-up of patients with adolescent idiopathic scoliosis treated conservatively: an analysis of the clinical value of progression. *J Pediatr Orthop*. 1990;10:48-52.

18. Peltonen J, Poussa M, Ylikoski M. Three-year results of bracing in scoliosis. *Acta Orthop Scand*. 1988;59:487-490.

19. Rowe DE, Bernstein SM, Riddick MF, Adler F, Emans JB, Gardner-Bonneau D. A meta-analysis of the efficacy of nonoperative treatments for idiopathic scoliosis. *J Bone Joint Surg [Am]*. 1997;79:664-674.

20. Winter RB, Lonstein JE, Drogt J, Noren CA. The effectiveness of bracing in the nonoperative treatment of idiopathic scoliosis. *Spine*. 1986;11:790-791.

21. Carter VM, Fasen JM, Roman JM, Hayes KW, Petersen CM. The effect of a soft collar, used as normally recommended or reversed, on three planes of cervical range of motion. *J Orthop Sports Phys Ther*. 1996;23:209-215.

22. Kaufman BS, Lunsford TR, Lunsford BR, Lance LL. Comparison of three prefabricated cervical collars. *Orthotics and Prosthetics*. 1986;39:21-28.

23. Althoff B, Goldie IF. Cervical collars in rheumatoid atlanto-axial subluxation: a radiographic comparison. *Ann Rheum Dis*. 1980;39:485-489.

24. Lunsford TR, Davidson M, Lunsford BR. The effectiveness of four contemporary cervical orthoses in restricting cervical motion. *Journal of Prosthetics and Orthotics*. 1994;6:93-99.

25. Sandler AJ, Dvorak J, Humke T, Grob D, Daniels W. The effectiveness of several cervical orthoses: an in vivo comparison of the mechanical stability provided by several widely used models. *Spine*. 1996;21:1624-1629.

26. Catipovic RM, Tittle LA, Mollendorf JC. A new cervical-thoracic orthosis: clinical report of seven cases. *Journal of Prosthetics and Orthotics.* 1998;10:33-36.

27. Sharpe KP, Rao S, Ziogas A. Evaluation of the effectiveness of the Minerva cervicothoracic orthosis. *Spine.* 1995;20:1475-1479.

28. Richardson JK, Ross ADM, Riley B, Rhodes RL. Halo vest effect on balance. *Arch Phys Med Rehabil.* 2000;81:255-257.

RECOMMENDED READING

1. Bassett GS, Bunnell WP, MacEwen GD. Treatment of idiopathic scoliosis with the Wilmington brace. *J Bone Joint Surg [Am].* 1986;68:602-605.

2. Beavis A. Cervical orthoses. *Prosthet Orthot Int.* 1989;13:6-13.

3. Cassella MC, Hall JE. Current treatment approaches in the nonoperative and operative management of adolescent idiopathic scoliosis. *Phys Ther.* 1991;71:897-909.

4. Emans JB, Kaelin A, Bancel P, et al. The Boston bracing system for idiopathic scoliosis: follow-up results in 295 patients. *Spine.* 1986;11:792-801.

5. Price CT, Scott DS, Reed FE, Riddick MF. Nighttime bracing for adolescent idiopathic scoliosis with the Charleston bending brace: preliminary report. *Spine.* 1990;15:1294-1299.

CASE STUDIES

For the following cases, select an appropriate orthosis, establish long- and short-term treatment goals, and develop a treatment plan.

- FC is a 46-year-old bookkeeper who did an unaccustomed amount of gardening. He awoke the next morning with severe low back pain with radiation to the left buttock and down the back of the left leg. He complains of pain when bending forward or to the left, as well as on straight leg raising and resisted left hip adduction and flexion. In supine, he has pain upon pressure on the anterior superior iliac spines bilaterally. On sidelying on the right, pain occurs on the left iliac crest. In prone, pressure on the sacrum is painful. He reports paresthesia in his left foot, especially the heel. The patella tendon and Achilles' tendon reflexes are normal, as is muscle strength.

- RK is a 72-year-old museum volunteer with severe osteoporosis. She reports that she is 2 inches shorter than she was when she was in her 20s and that her dresses no longer fit straight on her torso. She has mild left thoracic, right lumbar kyphoscoliosis, and pelvic obliquity. Recently, she developed pain in the midthorax.

- AN is a 14-year-old student with 30-degree idiopathic right thoracic, left lumbar scoliosis, and pelvic obliquity with the left hip higher than the right. Leg lengths are equal. She was so concerned about her appearance that she started crying when her physician recommended an orthosis.

- MT is a 35-year-old attorney who sustained a hyperextension injury when his car was struck from the rear 6 weeks ago. Radiographs show no fractures. He reports that all neck motions are painful, especially neck extension. Passive motion is limited in neck extension and lateral rotation to both sides.

- LR is a 67-year-old seamstress who was attacked by a man who was trying to steal her purse. The assailant pushed her violently onto some concrete steps. At the hospital she was diagnosed with a C5 fracture. Her neck was surgically stabilized and she was placed in halo traction for 8 weeks. The fracture has healed, and the traction has been removed. She has very limited active motion in her neck and complains of pain radiating down her left arm to the wrist. The left biceps reflex is decreased. She has fair strength in her left rotator cuff muscles, biceps, brachialis, brachioradialis, deltoids, teres major, and rhomboids. All other muscle groups have normal strength.

POINT/COUNTERPOINT

BL is a 27-year-old teacher who is in the sixth month of her first pregnancy. She has been experiencing severe back pain that radiates into her left buttock and down the posterior aspect of her left leg to the heel. Pain is elicited with trunk flexion, left straight leg raising, lateral flexion to the left, pressure on the sacrum with the patient prone, and pressure on the anterior superior iliac spines bilaterally with the patient supine. Pain is relieved with pressure on the iliac crest with the patient sidelying on the right side. The right leg is 3 cm longer than the left one when the patient is supine, but the lower extremities are equal in length when she sits with the legs extended.

JOAN SAYS	JAN SAYS

Orthotic Prescription

Ligamentous laxity and the increasing abdominal weight are major factors contributing to her pain. Rather than the sacroiliac belt, I suggest a lumbosacral corset with elastic abdominal support and side-laced panels to accommodate the enlarging abdomen. The corset will distribute force over a larger area of the torso and thus should be more comfortable.

I recommend the least restrictive orthosis that will stabilize the pelvic girdle as the hormonal changes occurring during pregnancy cause ligamentous laxity. Thus, a sacroiliac belt should be adequate to relieve her pain.

Long-Term Goals

I am concerned about controlling pain so that she can continue teaching for another 2 months in reasonable comfort. I am also considering her postpartum health:
- Reduce pain
- Determine whether leg-length discrepancy exists; if so, determine the extent to which it contributes to pain

In order to keep this patient comfortable during her pregnancy, I suggest:
- Resolve pain to a manageable level
- Resolve leg-length discrepancy

Short-Term Goals

- Reduce pain by at least two points in 2 weeks
- Evaluate leg lengths in standing by using lift blocks under the left foot
- Achieve independent donning of the orthosis

- Reduce pain by two points on the verbal pain scale in 2 weeks
- Further investigate causes of leg-length discrepancy

JOAN SAYS	JAN SAYS

Treatment Plan

- Teach the patient to don the orthosis correctly, emphasizing the need to fasten the corset from the inferior portion upward. Alert the patient to methods of skin inspection using a hand-held mirror.
- Heat and massage to alleviate pain. Create a home program so that patient can apply a heating pad safely and can massage the sacroiliac region herself.
- Gentle stretching exercise to the low back.
- Select chair and bed positions that are most comfortable.

- Spinal mobilization to reduce back pain.
- Home exercise program for back and sacroiliac stabilization with exercises in quadruped and cat back position, including limb lifts and postural stability exercises.
- Positioning with pillows for better support in sitting, sidelying, and supine.
- Moist heat, as tolerated, to the sacroiliac region.
- Instruct her husband in low back massage.
- Gait analysis to assess presence and possible effect of leg-length discrepancy and possible need for orthotic modification of shoes.

Chapter 8

Upper-Limb Orthoses

Take a tender little hand,
Fringed with dainty fingerettes,
Press it—in parenthesis—
Take all these, you lucky man.
William Schwenk Gilbert, The Gondoliers

Orthoses for the upper limb range from appliances for the shoulder, including slings and rigid orthoses, to elbow orthoses, to a very wide variety of hand and wrist-hand devices. Those intended for relatively short-term use are often referred to as *splints*.

In addition to considering orthoses according to the portion of the upper limb that is braced, one may also classify devices with regard to primary function, namely assistive or substitutive, protective, or corrective. Assistive and substitutive orthoses are indicated for patients with paralysis; the devices augment residual motor power or substitute mechanical joint motion and stabilization for absent anatomical function. Protective orthoses either shield the affected joint from the likelihood of developing contracture, as is the case with burns, or reduce painful motion, often required with arthritis. Corrective orthoses are used to increase joint range of motion in the presence of dermal or capsular contracture.

Gadget tolerance (ie, the patient's willingness to wear orthoses) is relevant for all orthoses, but it is particularly important with regard to hand and wrist-hand orthoses. These devices are always visible. While they should benefit the patient, they are likely to frustrate the person during the performance of daily activities if they are cumbersome, uncomfortable, or cover sensate portions of the hand.

HAND AND WRIST-HAND ORTHOSES

Assistive and substitutive hand orthoses (HOs) and wrist-hand orthoses (WHOs) are widely used in rehabilitation.[1,2] Although many designs were developed for patients who had contracted poliomyelitis, the orthoses are currently prescribed primarily for individuals with central and peripheral neuropathies. Assistive orthoses position the hand so that the patient can make maximum use of residual motor power. Substitutive orthoses enable the patient to achieve prehension by moving the wrist or a more proximal body segment to cause finger movement.

Assistive Orthoses

Of the assistive HOs, the basic opponens orthosis (Figures 8-1a and 8-1b) is one of the simplest. Formerly called the short opponens splint, it keeps the thumb pad beneath the palmar surfaces of the index and middle fingers, assisting the patient to use residual motor power to achieve palmar prehension.

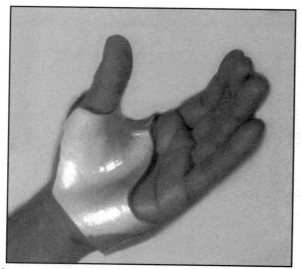

Figure 8-1a. Basic opponens orthosis—plastic.

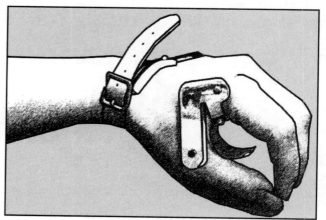

Figure 8-1b. Basic opponens orthosis—aluminum.

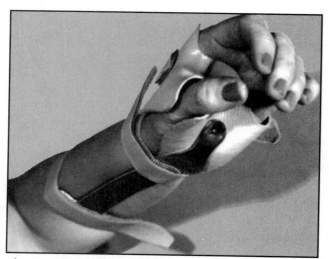

Figure 8-2. Opponens orthosis with wrist control (reproduced from American Academy of Orthopaedic Sugeons. *Atlas of Orthotics: Biomechanical Principles and Application.* 2nd ed. Philadelphia, PA: W. B. Saunders; 1985:165 with permission of W. B. Saunders Company).

Its dorsal and palmar bars support the transverse palmar arch, protecting it from flattening. The abduction bar keeps the thumb abducted, preventing thenar web contracture and placing the thumb in a suitable position for opposition. The opponens bar prevents the first metatarsal from migrating to the plane of the other fingers.[3] This orthosis is useful for the patient with median neuropathy who is in jeopardy of developing thenar contracture and a flat hand posture, and who needs assistance for prehension.

A forearm bar may be added to the basic opponens orthosis to create the opponens wrist-hand orthosis with wrist control (Figure 8-2), also known as the long opponens splint. The forearm bar may be located on the palmar, dorsal, radial, or ulnar aspect of the wrist and forearm. The forearm bar maintains the wrist in a fixed position, preventing the hand from dropping into palmar flexion.

Another addition to the basic opponens orthosis is a metacarpophalangeal extension stop (Figure 8-3). The stop, sometimes called a lumbrical bar, is secured to the palmar bar and applies palmarward force to the proximal phalanges to resist metacarpophalangeal hyperextension. This component protects the hand from forming claw hand deformity, which is a risk in the presence of ulnar or combined median and ulnar neuropathy, and thereby aids prehension.

Another assistive WHO is the wrist flexion control WHO (Figure 8-4), also called a cock-up splint. This design features a palmar hand bar and a palmar forearm bar with straps to secure the orthosis to the limb. The orthosis prevents the wrist from dropping into inadvertent palmar flexion seen in radial neuropathy, thereby assisting the median and ulnarly innervated muscles, which are placed in a more functional position. The same orthosis is often used to protect the wrist from repetitive motion strain, as experienced by keyboard operators.

Substitutive Orthoses

Prehension orthoses are examples of substitutive appliances. They are especially suited to the patient with tetraplegia. The orthoses enable the wearer to grasp, hold, and release an object voluntarily. The wrist-driven prehension WHO (Figure 8-5) originated as the flexor hinge orthosis because it has a

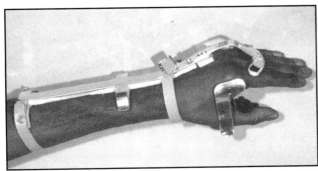

Figure 8-3. Opponens orthosis with metacarpophalangeal extension stop.

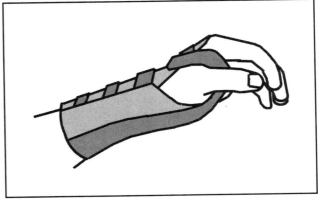

Figure 8-4. Wrist flexion control orthosis.

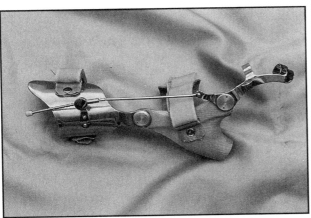

Figure 8-5. Wrist-driven prehension orthosis.

hinged linkage between the forearm bar and the finger stabilizers. The orthosis includes a bar and band that stabilize the first interphalangeal joint and a separate bar and band unit that prevents motion of the second and third proximal and distal interphalangeal joints. The two stabilizers pivot on a palmar and dorsal hand bar assembly on the radial side of the second metacarpophalangeal joint. A second pivot is located at the junction between the hand and forearm bar at the wrist.

When the patient extends the wrist, the linkage causes the finger stabilizer to approach the thumb stabilizer, enabling grasp. The user must maintain active extension in order to retain the held object. Some prehension orthoses have a locking mechanism to relieve stress on the wrist extensors.

Release of the object occurs when the wearer relaxes the wrist extensors, allowing the wrist to flex passively.[4,5] The patient with C6 tetraplegia can use the orthosis only in the position of forearm pronation. If the forearm was supinated, the wearer could achieve grasp and holding but could not release the object voluntarily because the individual lacked control of the palmar flexors. Nevertheless, the wrist-

driven prehension WHO is a relatively useful device, facilitating hygiene, writing, and feeding.

Most wrist-driven prehension orthoses have a mechanism that enables the wearer to select the size of grasp. For grasping a piece of paper, the wearer would adjust the mechanism so that a small arc of wrist motion achieved finger closure. For grasping a thicker object, the wearer would adjust the mechanism so that the same small arc of wrist extension achieved wider closure.

The patient with C4 or C5 tetraplegia lacks sufficient control of the wrist extensors and consequently requires another version of prehension orthosis. The electrically-driven prehension WHO is sometimes prescribed. The rigid parts of the orthosis are similar to those of the wrist-driven model; however, instead of a linkage between hand and forearm components, the electrically driven orthosis has a steel cable secured to the finger stabilizer. The proximal end of the cable terminates in a rod linked to a battery-operated motor. To achieve grasp, the patient moves an actuator, usually located over the contralateral shoulder, to trigger a microswitch. The switch turns on the motor, which pulls the cable proximally. Cable movement causes the finger stabilizer to approach the thumb stabilizer. Holding occurs when the patient causes the motor to stall. Release is attained by voluntary shoulder pressure on a second microswitch in the actuator. The latter reverses the direction of the motor, relieving tension on the cable. A spring located on the finger stabilizer is then able to recoil, opening the fingers. Usually a relatively large arc of shoulder elevation causes grasp and a smaller arc triggers the releasing microswitch.

The battery and motor are relatively heavy and bulky but are easily transported on a wheelchair. The individual who has hand paralysis and is ambulatory would not be a candidate for an electrically driven orthosis. As with all battery-powered motors, the

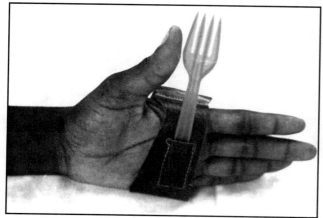

Figure 8-6. Utensil holder.

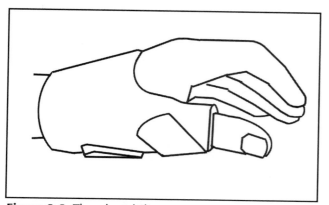

Figure 8-8. Thumb stabilizer.

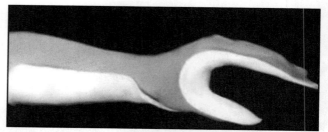

Figure 8-7. Wrist-hand stabilizer without straps.

slender can have an adapter attached to it so that it can fit snugly in the pocket.

Protective Orthoses

Many protective WHOs are mass-produced, although nearly all the designs can be custom-made of plaster of Paris or plastic sheeting.

The wrist-hand stabilizer orthosis (Figure 8-7), also termed a resting splint, is a sheet of semirigid plastic placed on the palmar surface of the hand and forearm.[6-8] The sheet extends from the distal tips of the fingers to the middle third of the forearm and is curved to support the palmar arch and cradle the forearm. Straps secure the plastic to the hand and forearm. Some stabilizers include a thumb component to prevent motion of that digit. The stabilizer is widely used by patients with exacerbation of rheumatoid arthritis and those with burns who are vulnerable to flexion contractures.

In a prospective randomized study of patients who had carpal tunnel syndrome, those who wore a wrist-hand stabilizer full-time achieved reduction of functional deficits and improved response to nerve conduction studies as compared with those who wore the same type of orthosis only at night.[9]

A thumb stabilizer (Figure 8-8) prevents movement of the first interphalangeal and metacarpophalangeal joints. The orthosis consists of a longitudinal bar along the length of the thumb with stabilizing straps or a sleeve on the thumb and a strap around the hand.

A finger stabilizer (Figure 8-9) is used for the patient with boutonniere deformity, which is persistent flexion of the proximal interphalangeal joint. It includes a band that applies palmarly directed force at the proximal interphalangeal joint. Two bands that apply dorsally directed forces to the proximal and middle phalanges oppose the force.

Corrective Orthoses

Corrective orthoses apply a low, constant force with appropriate counterforces to reduce contrac-

battery in the orthosis must be recharged periodically. Many patients eventually opt for a much simpler orthosis to facilitate grasp, eliminating the necessity of battery charging and wearing a rather cumbersome appliance.

The utensil holder (Figure 8-6) is an orthosis, usually mass-produced, that consists of a spring clip or elastic webbing around the circumference of the palm. The palmar side of the clip has a slim leather pocket into which one may place a pen, spoon handle, or other objects of appropriate size. It is sometimes called a universal cuff. The orthosis may have a forearm bar to prevent unwanted wrist motion so that the hand remains in a more functional position. Grasping is achieved by inserting an object or a handle into the pocket. Patients often accomplish this by holding the object with the teeth and directing it into the pocket. Alternatively, an attendant may place an object in the pocket. The pocket stabilizes the object, holding it in place. Release requires removing the object from the pocket with the teeth or other means. An object that is too large to fit into the pocket or too

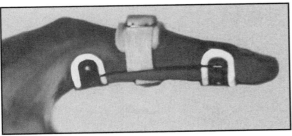

Figure 8-9. Finger stabilizer.

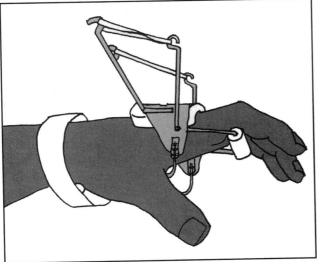

Figure 8-11. Finger extensor orthosis.

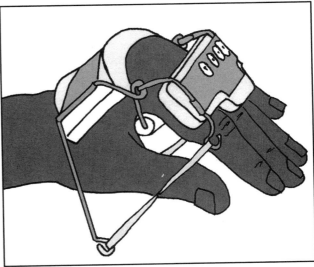

Figure 8-10. Finger flexor orthosis.

FOREARM AND ELBOW ORTHOSES

As a group, elbow and forearm orthoses are less frequently prescribed. Nevertheless, some patients benefit from protective or corrective elbow orthoses; very few tolerate assistive or substitutive elbow orthoses.

Protective and Corrective Orthoses

Forearm cuffs (Figure 8-12) are readily available to reduce stress on forearm extensors for patients who have lateral epicondylitis, commonly termed "tennis elbow." The typical cuff is made of sturdy fabric with a hook-and-pile closure.[11,12] Some cuffs have reinforcing bars.

In the presence of elbow flexion contracture, the elbow extensor orthosis (Figure 8-13) can effectively increase elbow excursion if the patient wears the appliance continuously. Both mass-produced and custom-made orthoses are available. Regardless of their source, however, all have the same three-point pressure system, namely anteriorly directed force in the vicinity of the olecranon and posteriorly directed counterforces at the distal forearm and proximal upper arm. Most models have an adjustable mechanism that permits the clinician to elongate the distance between the forearm and upper arm as the contracture reduces. Others have a spring mechanism that is designed to maintain maximum separation between the cuffs. In the absence of an adjustable joint or spring, the orthosis is designed to be remolded periodically as the contracture reduces.

ture. Such appliances are usually factory-made but can also be custom-made. The patient who has a flat hand with extension contractures of the metacarpophalangeal joints may be fitted with a finger flexor HO (Figure 8-10), also known as a knuckle bender. It has a dorsally located plate over the metacarpals and another plate over the proximal phalanges linked to a palmar rod. Springs or rubber bands apply tensile force to the orthosis. If worn for a sufficient period of time, the orthosis will cause the metacarpophalangeal joints to yield. Care must be taken, however, to avoid undue pressure on the skin.

The finger extensor orthosis (Figure 8-11), also called the reverse knuckle bender, has an opposite force system, namely a palmarly located bar linked to two dorsal bars. Rubber bands or springs exert tension. Versions of these corrective orthoses are available to correct extension and flexion deformities of the interphalangeal joints. Neuromuscular electrical stimulation to forearm musculature, combined with a corrective WHO, reduces spasticity in children with cerebral palsy.[10]

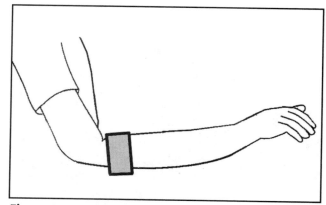

Figure 8-12. Forearm cuff.

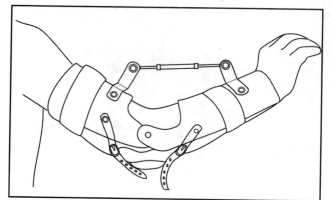

Figure 8-13. Elbow extensor orthosis.

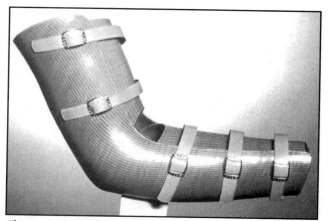

Figure 8-14. Elbow stabilizer.

Assistive and Substitutive Orthoses

Elbow assistive and substitutive orthoses are intended for patients who have paralysis of the elbow flexors or extensors. Lacking voluntary control of the elbow, the individual would have a limited work area in which to use the naturally or orthotically powered hand. The simplest orthosis is the elbow stabilizer (Figure 8-14), which maintains the elbow in partial flexion and the forearm in moderate pronation. The orthosis places the hand in a position to perform tabletop functions. The orthosis does not have moving parts, making it durable and relatively inexpensive. The elbow, however, is kept at a flexed position, which is awkward when the individual walks or dons a jacket.

A more versatile orthosis is the elbow flexion-extension orthosis, which resembles a transhumeral prosthesis. The custom-made orthosis has a distal forearm cuff and a proximal upper arm cuff, as well as a harness that fits around the torso. A steel cable extends from the harness to the distal cuff. The patient achieves elbow flexion by exerting force on

the harness by voluntary shoulder flexion. The force causes the cable to reduce the distance between the distal and proximal cuffs. Some orthoses have an elbow lock, which relieves the patient of the need to maintain shoulder flexion in order to keep the elbow flexed. When the patient relaxes the shoulder flexors, gravity straightens the elbow. More complex versions of the orthosis are occasionally made. These may include a hydraulic or pneumatic cylinder, which facilitates elbow motion or may use myoelectric control. The latter version has skin electrodes placed over muscles, which the patient can control voluntarily. Muscular contraction is transmitted to a motor that activates the orthotic elbow hinge. Such orthoses are relatively heavy, very expensive, fragile, and require frequent recharging of the battery that powers the motor.

A new approach to improve grasp for children with spastic cerebral palsy involves an elbow-wrist-hand orthosis with neuromuscular electrical stimulation of the wrist extensors. Preliminary experience demonstrates improvement in wrist and hand posture and improved strength and control of grasp and release.[13]

SHOULDER ORTHOSES

Most shoulder orthoses protect the glenohumeral joint from subluxation, which usually occurs because the patient has flaccid hemiplegia or injury to the shoulder joint capsule.

Protective Orthoses

The simplest such orthosis is a sling, a widely used type of upper-limb orthosis. Although many designs have been created, the most common categories are single-strap, multiple-strap, and humeral cuff slings.

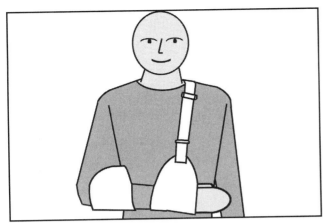

Figure 8-15. Single-strap sling.

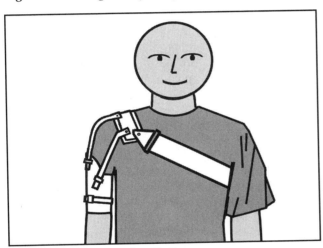

Figure 8-17. Humeral cuff sling.

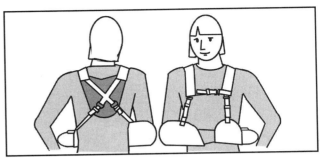

Figure 8-16. Multiple-strap sling.

Because it has one strap that lies vertically over the ipsilateral shoulder, the multiple-strap sling directly resists downward shoulder subluxation. As is true of single-strap slings, multiple-strap versions also support the weight of the forearm and hand to prevent the limb from swinging into objects. Both single- and multiple-strap slings keep the elbow flexed, which is a nuisance when the wearer dons a coat.

Humeral cuff slings (Figure 8-17) do not have a forearm support. Instead, they have a broad cuff that encircles the upper arm. Vertical straps extend from the anterior and posterior proximal margins of the cuff to a horizontal strap that encircles the chest. Some models have a pad over the shoulder to lessen pressure concentration. Humeral cuff slings resist shoulder subluxation without encumbering the elbow or forearm. Consequently, the wearer can conceal the sling under a shirt. One version of the humeral cuff sling has cuffs on both upper arms. The cuffs are jointed posteriorly by a strap. Tightening the strap causes both humeri to lodge firmly in their respective glenohumeral fossae.[15-18]

Corrective Orthoses

In addition to slings, shoulder orthoses also include appliances that have a jointed metal frame with cuffs and straps. Depending on the type of metal joint, these orthoses may either correct existing axillary contracture or substitute motion if the patient has paralysis of the shoulder in combination with distal weakness.

The shoulder abductor orthosis (Figure 8-18) is designed to correct axillary contracture by positioning the arm in the maximum degree of abduction that the patient can tolerate. If the arm is held in abduction, the orthosis is also called an airplane splint. If the forearm is kept vertically upward, the orthosis is sometimes referred to as the "Statue of Liberty" because the patient's arm is held in an upright position, similar to the posture of the torch-holding limb of the statue.

The typical single-strap sling (Figure 8-15) has a canvas forearm support to which is sewn a strap that is worn over the contralateral shoulder. The forearm support may be a continuous piece of fabric or may be divided into proximal and distal forearm sections. The single-strap sling supports the weight of the forearm, wrist, and hand, which may be particularly desirable in the presence of edema or a plaster cast. The sling resists shoulder subluxation in patients with flaccid paralysis of shoulder musculature. It is also useful to prevent a flail upper limb from swinging and inadvertently bumping into objects.[14] The single strap sling is easier to don than other models.

Multiple-strap slings (Figure 8-16) have two or more straps. Proximal and distal straps join the forearm support. The proximal strap passes over the ipsilateral shoulder, while the distal strap lies over the opposite shoulder. In back, the two straps may be sewn into an oblique strap that maintains the appropriate distance between the two vertical straps.

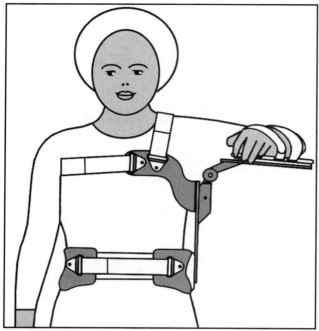

Figure 8-18. Shoulder abductor stabilizer.

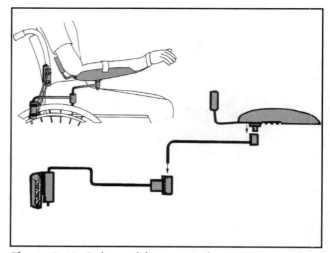

Figure 8-19. Balanced forearm orthosis.

Assistive Orthoses

Patients who retain function in the hand and elbow but have lost control of the shoulder will be able to make better use of the hand if the shoulder is stabilized. A shoulder stabilizer orthosis has a metal frame for the upper arm; the frame is joined to a trunk orthosis. The most common shoulder joint is a friction joint, which keeps the wearer's shoulder in the desired position.

When shoulder motion is desired, the most practical orthosis is the balanced forearm orthosis (BFO) (Figure 8-19). It is sometimes referred to as a "feeder" because it facilitates shoulder and elbow motions needed for feeding. This is a mass-produced appliance that is usually bolted to the wheelchair. The BFO consists of a proximal link, which fits into a ball-bearing receptacle attached to the wheelchair or other support, and a distal link, which fits into a second ball-bearing receptacle between the proximal and distal links. The distal link is attached to a pivoting rocker mechanism to which the forearm trough is screwed. By adjusting the tilt and rotational position of the proximal and distal links, one can assist or resist shoulder flexion, extension, and rotation.

The first mechanical principle that governs the BFO is the inclined plane. Objects move down a slope. For example, if the elbow extensors are weaker than the flexors, the proximal and distal links will be tilted so that they slope downward. They will assist elbow extension for reaching maneuvers but will require the patient to exert flexion force to return the forearm to the mouth. The second principle is that of the first-class lever exemplified by the action of the forearm trough. If the proximal portion of the trough is screwed into the pivoting mechanism, elbow extension is aided. Locating the screws toward the distal end of the trough assists elbow flexion.

The BFO is a relatively inexpensive orthosis that enables the user to move the arm horizontally and vertically. It is usually employed with a wheelchair to enable the patient with tetraplegia to accomplish many daily activities, such as feeding, facial hygiene, writing, keyboard operation, and painting if the patient retains natural or orthotically assisted prehension.

FABRICATION OPTIONS

Most mass-produced upper-limb orthoses are designed to be adjusted to fit the given patient. Adjustment may take the form of loosening or tightening straps or laces, adding or subtracting rubber bands or wires, or heating and bending plastic components.

HOs and WHOs, however, can be custom-made rather easily.[6] Clinicians who specialize in WHOs often select one or two materials from the wide range of thermoplastics to gain proficiency with molding them on the patient. The first step involves creating a paper pattern of the orthosis. One may drape paper towels on the hand, trimming the paper until a snug fit is achieved. Books of splint patterns[3,8,19] suggest basic designs. The pattern is then traced from the paper onto the plastic. The plastic is heated, in most cases in warm water, to the temperature specified by the manufacturer. Some plastics, particularly those made in open or closed cellular foam, need to be heated in an oven. While the plastic is heating, the clinician protects the patient's hand with a stockinette. When the plastic reaches a pliable state, it is trimmed along the traced lines, then molded over the body segment. Depending on the size of the splint, the clinician may hold the warm plastic in place or secure it with an elastic bandage until the plastic is cool. The final step involves finishing the edges and securing straps or other accessories.

If the thermoplastic was shaped in warm water, the patient must be cautioned to not immerse it in warm water, which would distort it. If a foam plastic was used, it should not be subjected to any fluid, which would collect in the cells. Directly formed plastics are also vulnerable to distortion if subjected to dry heat for an extended period (eg, one should not keep the splint in a car parked in a sunny location).

UPPER-LIMB ORTHOSIS EVALUATION: FINGER, WRIST-HAND, AND FOREARM ORTHOSES

- Orthosis is comfortable without excessive pressure, especially at bony prominences
- Mechanical joints are congruent with anatomical joints
- Palmar surfaces of the thumb and all fingers are uncovered, except for the wrist-hand stabilizer
- Opponens bar applies force over the first metacarpal and extends to the radial edge of the first metacarpal
- Thumb abduction bar maintains adequate thumb abduction without restricting the thumb interphalangeal joint or the index metacarpophalangeal joint
- Palmar and dorsal bars are shaped and located to support the transverse arch and to permit full opposition
- Metacarpophalangeal extension stop is shaped and located to prevent metacarpophalangeal hyperextension
- Assistive and substitutive orthoses should have the thumb and fingers positioned to provide opposition
- Wrist strap lies snugly between the bases of the metacarpals and the wrist crease without interfering with wrist motion
- Forearm bar stabilizes the wrist in the desired position

- Forearm bar does not restrict elbow motion
- Patient can open and close the fingers completely
- Patient can operate the control mechanism
- Patient has adequate pinch force
- Utensils are properly positioned and sufficiently stabilized in the utensil pocket

UPPER-LIMB ORTHOSIS EVALUATION: ELBOW AND SHOULDER ORTHOSES

- Orthosis is comfortable without excessive pressure, especially at bony prominences
- Mechanical joints are congruent with anatomical joints
- Forearm, elbow, and shoulder have intended range of motion
- Glenohumeral joint is well-supported
- Patient can operate the control mechanism

GUIDELINES FOR PRESCRIPTION

The following are biomechanical guidelines for prescribing upper-limb orthoses:
1. To maintain opposed position of the thumb, index, and middle fingers, particularly for patients with median neuropathy. Selection depends on the amount, if any, of additional motion restriction that may be beneficial.
   a. Basic opponens orthosis
   b. Opponens orthosis with wrist control
   c. Opponens orthosis with metacarpophalangeal extension stop
2. To prevent claw deformities of the fingers and to assist finger extension, particularly for patients with ulnar neuropathy or combined median-ulnar neuropathy. Selection depends on the amount, if any, of additional motion restriction that may be beneficial.
   a. Opponens orthosis with metacarpophalangeal extension stop
   b. Opponens orthosis with metacarpophalangeal extension stop and wrist control
3. To limit wrist palmar flexion, particularly for patients with radial neuropathy. Selection depends on the amount, if any, of additional motion restriction that may be beneficial.
   a. Wrist flexion control orthosis
   b. Opponens orthosis with wrist control

4. To enable prehension for patients who have finger paralysis but who retain fair plus or stronger wrist extensors, such as patients with C6 tetraplegia. Selection depends on the individual's gadget tolerance.

   a. Wrist-driven prehension orthosis

   b. Utensils with large handles

5. To enable prehension for patients who have hand and wrist paralysis, such as patients with C5 or higher tetraplegia. Selection depends on the individual's gadget tolerance.

   a. Electrically-driven prehension orthosis

   b. Passive prehension orthosis

   c. Utensil holder

6. To restrict motion of the wrist and hand, particularly for patients with painful arthritis or carpal tunnel syndrome.

   a. Wrist-hand stabilizer

7. To restrict motion of the first interphalangeal and metacarpophalangeal joints.

   a. Thumb stabilizer

8. To restrict finger motion.

   a. Finger stabilizer

9. To increase flexion of the metacarpophalangeal joints.

   a. Finger flexor orthosis (knuckle bender)

10. To increase extension of the metacarpophalangeal joints.

   a. Finger extensor orthosis (reverse knuckle bender)

11. To reduce stress on the forearm extensors, particularly for patients with lateral epicondylitis.

   a. Forearm cuff

12. To increase elbow extension by applying anteriorly directed force to the olecranon and posteriorly directed forces proximal and distal to the elbow.

   a. Elbow extensor orthosis

13. To assist upper-limb function in the presence of elbow weakness. Selection depends on the individual's gadget tolerance.

   a. Elbow stabilizer

   b. Elbow orthosis with hydraulically, electrically, or cable-controlled hinge

14. To reduce stress on the shoulder joint. Selection depends on the individual's gadget tolerance.

   a. Single-strap sling

   b. Multiple-strap sling

   c. Humeral cuff sling

15. To increase shoulder flexion and abduction or prevent contracture.

   a. Shoulder orthosis with adjustable hinge

16. To assist shoulder and elbow motion.

   a. Balanced forearm orthosis

SUMMARY

Upper-limb orthoses may assist or substitute motion, protect the segment from developing contracture, reduce painful motion, or correct contractures. HOs include the basic opponens orthosis, which assists the patient with median neuropathy by maintaining the transverse palmar arch, keeping the thumb abducted and in optimal position for prehension. A forearm bar may be added to this orthosis, which becomes a WHO. A metacarpophalangeal extension stop added to the orthosis applies palmarward force to the proximal phalanges, preventing claw hand deformity, as might develop with ulnar or combined median and ulnar neuropathy. The wrist flexion control orthosis prevents wrist drop, which might occur with radial lesion. Prehension orthoses are designed for patients with tetraplegia. The wrist-driven prehension orthosis enables the patient to achieve grasp by active wrist extension. Orthotic linkage draws the index and middle fingers toward the thumb. Relaxing the extensors allows gravity to open the orthosis so that the patient can release the held object. The person who cannot actively extend the wrist may benefit from an electrically-driven prehension orthosis or a utensil holder.

Protective WHOs include the thumb stabilizer and the wrist-hand stabilizer. Corrective orthoses, such as the flexor WHO, apply low, constant force to reduce contractures.

A forearm cuff orthosis may remind the patient who has lateral epicondylitis not to move through a painful arc of motion. An extensor elbow orthosis can reduce a flexion contracture. Assistive and substitutive elbow orthoses include the elbow stabilizer and the cable-operated elbow orthosis.

Slings are a popular type of shoulder orthosis and include single-strap and multiple-strap versions, as well as the humeral cuff designs. Jointed metal shoulder orthoses correct axillary contracture or substitute for shoulder motion in the presence of paralysis. The balanced forearm orthosis is a versatile orthosis that assists shoulder and elbow motion.

Orthoses may be mass-produced or custom-made with plastics that are designed to be formed directly on the patient.

THOUGHT QUESTIONS

1. Describe a WHO that would enable a butcher who exhibits wrist-drop following radial neuropathy to return to work while the injury heals.

2. Diagram the force system that would restrict progression of swan-neck deformity secondary to rheumatoid arthritis.

3. What is the functional position of the hand for the patient with median neuropathy? What deformities would develop if the patient were not fitted with an appropriate orthosis?

4. Describe an orthosis that would enable a dentist with biceps brachii paralysis secondary to laceration of the musculocutaneous nerve to continue his practice.

5. Describe the characteristics of the ideal candidate for the wrist-driven prehension orthosis.

REFERENCES

1. Fess EE, Philips CA. *Hand Splinting: Principles and Methods*. 2nd ed. St. Louis, Mo: The CV Mosby Company; 1987.

2. Irani KD. Upper limb orthoses. In: Braddom RL, ed. *Physical Medicine and Rehabilitation*. Philadelphia, Pa: WB Saunders; 1996:321-332.

3. Malick MH. *Manual on Static Hand Splinting: New Materials and Techniques*. Pittsburgh, Pa: Harmarville Rehabilitation Center; 1972.

4. Makaran JE, Dittmer DK, Buchal RO, MacArthur DE. The SMART wrist-hand orthosis (WHO) for quadriplegic patients. *Journal of Prosthetics and Orthotics*. 1993;5:73-76.

5. Malick MH, Meyer CMH. *Manual on Management of the Quadriplegic Upper Extremity*. Pittsburgh, Pa: Harmarville Rehabilitation Center; 1978.

6. McKee P, Morgan L. *Orthotics in Rehabilitation: Splinting the Hand and Body*. Philadelphia, Pa: FA Davis; 1998.

7. Tenney CG, Lisak JM. *Atlas of Hand Splinting*. Boston, Mass: Little, Brown, and Company; 1986.

8. Wilton JC. *Hand Splinting: Principles of Design and Fabrication*. Philadelphia, Pa: WB Saunders; 1997.

9. Walker WC, Metzler M, Cifu DX, Swartz Z. Neural wrist splinting in carpal tunnel syndrome: a comparison of night-one versus full-time wear instructions. *Arch Phys Med Rehabil*. 2000;81:424-429.

10. Scheker LR, Chesher SP, Ramirez S. Neuromuscular electrical stimulation and dynamic bracing as a treatment for upper-extremity spasticity in children with cerebral palsy. *J Hand Surg [Br]*. 1999;24:226-232.

11. Snyder-Mackler L, Epler M. Effect of standard and Aircast tennis elbow bands on integrated electromyography of forearm extensor musculature proximal to the bands. *Am J Sports Med*. 1989;17:278-281.

12. Wuori JL, Overend TJ, Kramer JF, MacDermid J. Strength and pain measures associated with lateral epicondylitis bracing. *Arch Phys Med Rehabil*. 1998;79:832-837.

13. Kleinert R. Neuromuscular electrical stimulation and dynamic bracing as a treatment for upper-extremity spasticity in children with cerebral palsy. *J Hand Surg [Br]*. 1999;24:226-232.

14. Rajaram Y, Holtz M. Shoulder forearm support for the subluxed shoulder. *Arch Phys Med Rehabil*. 1985;66:191-192.

15. Brooke MM, de Lateur BJ, Diana-Rigby GC, Questad KA. Shoulder subluxation in hemiplegia: effects of three different supports. *Arch Phys Med Rehabil*. 1991;72:582-586.

16. Claus SW, Godfrey KJ. A new distal support sling for the hemiplegic patient. *Am J Occup Ther*. 1985;39:536-537.

17. Idank DM, Zorowitz RD, Ikai T, Hughes MB, Johnston MV. Shoulder subluxation after stroke: a pilot study comparing four slings. *Arch Phys Med Rehabil*. 1993;74:12-35.

18. Zorowitz RD, Idank D, Ikai T, Hughes MB, Johnston MV. Shoulder subluxation after stroke: a comparison of four supports. *Arch Phys Med Rehabil*. 1995;76:763-771.

19. Ziegler EM. *Current Concepts in Orthotics: A Diagnosis-Related Approach to Splinting*. Minneapolis, Minn: Rolyan Medical Products; 1984.

CASE STUDIES

For the following cases, select an appropriate orthosis, establish long- and short-term goals, and develop a treatment plan.

- RM is a 68-year-old grandmother with severe rheumatoid arthritis. She has ulnar deviation of the metacarpophalangeal joints of both hands. She has severe pain in these joints and reports difficulty using chop sticks, which are the utensils she has used all her life for eating and cooking. She says she is a restless sleeper and will sometimes roll on her hands and then awake in severe pain.

- NF is a 23-year-old financial analyst who sustained C6 spinal cord injury as a result of a diving accident. She has had spinal fusion and is paralyzed below the level of the lesion.

- SB is a 17-year-old student who sustained a brachial plexus injury during a basketball game when he went up for a lay-up and came down tangled with the rebounders. His radial nerve was avulsed at the brachial plexus. All associated sensory and motor function has been lost. His physician is concerned that SB may develop contractures while the nerve is healing.

- MA is a 38-year-old data-entry clerk. She complains of pain, burning, and tingling on the palmar aspect of her right palm; thumb, index, and middle fingers; and the medial aspect of the ring finger. She reports severe paresthesia at night that wakens her. Pain now interferes with her work.

POINT/COUNTERPOINT

PN, a 72-year-old knitting shop owner, had a right cerebrovascular accident and now has left hemiplegia. Her left hand is tightly fisted, is nonfunctional, and demonstrates hypersensitive palmar grasp reflex. When she walks, her left arm pulls into a flexor synergy with noticeable increase in muscle tone. Her left shoulder is subluxed. Pain in her left shoulder radiates down the arm.

JOAN SAYS	JAN SAYS

Orthotic Prescription

- Single-strap sling to prevent subluxation and to resist the tendency of the arm to swing uncontrollably during gait training. Alternative sling designs encase the shoulder but do not restrain the elbow or forearm; this design fosters retention of the humeral head in the glenoid fossa, reducing painful stress on the shoulder ligamentous capsule
- Wrist-hand stabilizer made of low-temperature thermoplastic. Initially, the orthosis will be fitted with the thumb in maximally tolerated abduction and metacarpophalangeal joints in maximum extension, without slipping into hyperextension. The orthosis should support the palmar arch
- Posterior leaf spring AFO with tennis shoe
- Cane

- Wrist-hand orthosis that holds the wrist in 30 degrees of wrist extension, 130 degrees of metacarpophalangeal flexion, and thumb in opposition to the index finger. Orthosis should not contact the palm but should provide support from the dorsal surface of the hand and forearm
- Single-strap sling to support the arm and prevent shoulder subluxation
- Appropriate tests and measures to determine ambulatory level

Long-Term Goals

- Reduce pain in the shoulder
- Prevent contractures in the hand, elbow, and shoulder
- Achieve independence in orthotic donning
- Achieve independence in daily activities, including dressing, grooming, feeding, toileting, household ambulation, and wheelchair management

- Reduce pain in the arm
- Maintain sufficient range of motion in the left hand for hygiene
- Achieve independence in functional activities using one-handed techniques
- Achieve independence in orthotic management

| JOAN SAYS | JAN SAYS |

Short-Term Goals

- Don orthoses with minimal verbal cuing
- Instruct family member to observe whether the patient wears orthosis correctly
- Maintain maximum range of motion in all upper- and lower-limb joints
- Achieve safe transfer from wheelchair to toilet and other seats
- Achieve household ambulation
- Reevaluate fit of wrist-hand orthosis weekly and remold it to increase passive range of motion and prevent maceration of the skin

- Don orthoses with verbal cuing
- Self-applied range-of-motion exercises of the left arm with verbal cuing
- Perform self-care activities, including dressing, feeding, wheelchair management using one-handed techniques, and verbal cuing

Treatment Plan

- Teach the patient, with or without assistance from a family member, to don the orthosis
- Teach the patient how to propel wheelchair using the right hand and foot
- Teach the patient how to accomplish daily activities using the right hand
- Teach the patient and family members techniques for maintaining and increasing passive joint mobility in the left upper and lower limbs
- Arrange for weekly manicure to prevent the patient's fingernails from injuring her palm

- Orthotic training with the wrist-hand orthosis and sling
- Wheelchair management using one-handed techniques
- Activities of daily living training using one-handed techniques
- Instruction in range-of-motion exercises of the left arm that the patient can perform herself

Chapter 9

Orthoses for Burns and Other Soft Tissue Disorders

"The nurse... removed a small rectangular mirror... [and] brought it to George... The face that looked back at him... was not a face at all. It was a mask... George Bennett had been erased."
Milwaukee Journal Sentinel

INTRODUCTION

Orthoses can be used temporarily as part of the rehabilitation program for patients with burns or soft tissue disorders associated with neuromuscular pathology. Splints, positioning devices, and pressure garments can be instrumental in managing hypertrophic scarring and soft tissue adhesions. Clinicians should set goals with their patients that focus on functional activities at the highest level of independence. Orthoses can be very effective in helping patients achieve their goals if the appliances are part of a comprehensive rehabilitation program.

The hand is the most common area for splinting because it has many joints, a complex surface contour, minimal blood supply, and must function in numerous fine and gross tasks. A variety of hand orthoses address these demands. Other areas that are commonly splinted include the wrist, elbow, axilla, neck, ankle, and knee. These regions are at high risk for developing soft tissue contractures and, in the presence of burns, hypertrophic scarring.

Mass-produced orthoses for soft tissue disorders usually have hook-and-pile closures or zippers, enabling easy opening for wound inspection. They may have removable, washable linings and may be constructed of porous fabrics. Designs may include features that minimize pressure over bony prominences and maintain joint range of motion. Options on foot and ankle orthoses include high-traction soles to facilitate transfers and ambulation.

ORTHOSES FOR BURN MANAGEMENT

Management Issues

In contemporary practice, splint usage is rather sparing and selective. Individuals with partial-thickness burns usually receive splints when contractures start developing, after skin grafting, or following reconstructive surgery. Minimal encumbrance by restrictive equipment maximizes the patient's freedom of movement and the effectiveness of soft tissue care.[1-3]

Purposes of orthoses include managing scars, preventing deformity, protecting injured parts, and promoting function.

Managing Scars

Severe wounds resulting from deep partial-thickness and full-thickness burns proliferate granulation tissue as part of the healing process. Without proper management, cells laid down during the granulation phase will mature into a thick mass of tissue that is fragile, inflexible, and unsightly. Judiciously applied pressure can control the deposition of granulation tissue to prevent excessive scarring.[4-7]

Preventing Deformity

Burns, especially those that cause full-thickness wounds, tend to heal with excessive scarring unless collagen deposition is adequately controlled. If a burn occurs over a body part that normally has considerable mobility, excessive scarring will restrict motion, cause deformity, and impair function. For example, a full-thickness burn to the palmar aspect of the hand and fingers can result in severe flexion contractures, producing a fisted, nonfunctional hand. A goal of treatment would be to prevent deformity by maintaining good alignment of the fingers and hand. Functional splints would be an appropriate intervention.[8,9]

Protecting Injured Parts

Severe burns may destroy sensory nerve endings, depriving the patient of protective sensation. For example, a person who cannot distinguish hot and cold materials risks secondary thermal injury. With impaired proprioception and kinesthesia, a body part can get bruised or lacerated during the course of normal activities. A well-fitted orthosis protects the body from further trauma.

Promoting Function

Damaged skin, tendons, ligaments, nerves, and muscles may interfere with the patient's ability to transfer, ambulate, or perform other activities of daily living. Functional orthoses can help the patient achieve a maximal level of independent functioning while damaged structures heal.

Types of Orthoses

Pressure Garments

To control granulation and to prevent hypertrophic scarring, clinicians use custom-made, total-contact garments made of elastic fabric. They surround injured tissues to influence the regrowth of skin. For example, patients with burned hands may wear gauntlets or gloves (Figure 9-1). A well-designed pressure garment controls pain, provides a cosmetically acceptable cover over the burned area,

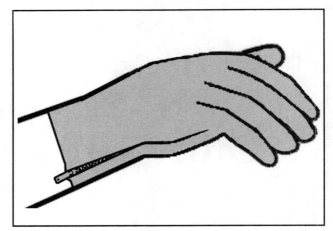

Figure 9-1. Elastic gauntlet.

protects against secondary trauma, and fosters a more functional outcome.[10]

Pressure garments present some difficulties. Many are difficult to don and doff independently, so patients may need assistance in dressing. They need at least two sets of garments so that one can be worn while a second is being laundered. The tight weave of the fabric inhibits ventilation, so patients may find the garments hot and uncomfortable. Each garment is made for a specific volume of tissue, so a garment will not be continuously effective in areas that are prone to fluctuating volume. The pressure gradient varies from one product to another,[11,12] making it difficult to assess the therapeutic effect of a specific garment.

Static Splints

Many orthoses can be categorized as static splints. They are usually made from sheet or foam plastic and are used most frequently for areas that have considerable mobility, such as the hand, neck, axilla, foot, and knee (Figures 9-2a and 9-2b). They are used to maintain joint alignment and protect the part from further trauma. Static splints hold a body part in one position.

For individuals with joint contractures, range of motion can be increased in two ways. One approach is to design static splints that can be remolded and thereby readjusted. These splints have no moving parts, have sleek trimlines, and are relatively lightweight. Unfortunately, the splinting material may weaken after repeated remolding so the appliance may lose effectiveness. The second approach employs a built-in mechanism for progressive serial splinting (Figure 9-3). The apparatus may be a strap, cord, or turnbuckle. This alternative adds to the weight, bulk, complexity, and cost of the appliances.

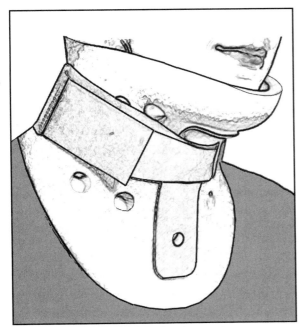

Figure 9-2a. Static splint for the neck.

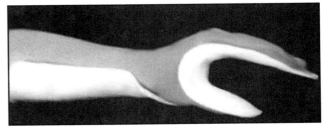

Figure 9-2b. Static splint for the the wrist. The wrist splint can be heated and remolded to accommodate a reduction in joint contracture. The straps will be added.

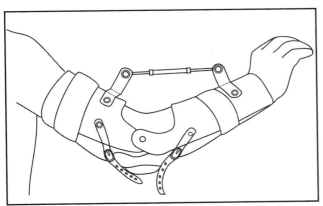

Figure 9-3. Progressive serial static splint for the elbow with a turnbuckle mechanism.

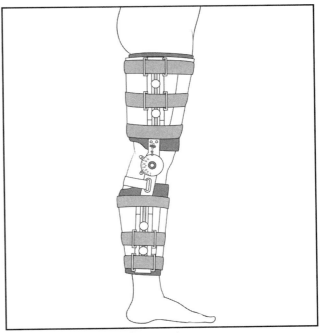

Figure 9-4. Dynamic knee splint.

Progressive serial splinting requires patient compliance and is contraindicated for uncooperative individuals or those with severe cognitive impairments.

Dynamic Splints

Devices that permit wearers to move within a controlled excursion are called dynamic splints (Figure 9-4). These orthoses enable individuals to increase joint range of motion. They also strengthen specific muscles by offering resistance. Corrective forces are exerted by elastic bands, wire springs, or fabric strips that are attached to the frame of the splint or are fastened to projections or extensions of the orthosis, called outriggers. Individuals should use dynamic splints as part of exercise regimens.

Positioning Splints

Orthoses can be used to position body parts to prevent joint contractures. As a general rule, positioning splints hold the body part in a position opposite to the most likely position of contracture and deformity. For example, if a patient sustains burns to the antecubital fossa of the elbow, the joint elbow is likely to develop a flexion contracture. The splint holds the elbow extended. Table 9-1 indicates the most commonly involved body parts, together with their position of likely contracture, and the recommended splinting position. Positioning splints are most commonly used for body parts that normally have increased mobility and with burns of major severity. Thus, areas with full-thickness burns and deep partial-thickness burns are more frequently splinted than are regions with superficial partial-thickness burns.

TABLE 9-1

Joint Positions for Patients with Burns

Body Segment	Position of Usual Deformity	Corrected Position	Orthotic/Positioning Implications
Neck	Flexion and rotation toward burned side	Slight neck extension; no lateral rotation; encourage sleeping in supine	Towel roll under neck, Philadelphia collar, or resilient egg-crate mattress to hold head and neck in slight extension
Shoulder	Adduction with slight internal rotation, neutral flexion	Abduction to 90 degrees, neutral rotation, and slight flexion	Foam plastic wedge or airplane abduction splint; avoid any position that would impinge on the brachial plexus
Elbow	Elbow flexion and forearm pronation	Elbow fully extended, forearm supinated	Pillows or foam plastic to position elbow and forearm on bed; elbow extensor orthosis; sling suspension
Wrist	Palmar flexion with deviation toward burn site	Extension with neutral deviation	Low-temperature plastic static splint; can use fabric splint over elastic garment or wrap
Hand and fingers	Claw hand; MCP hyperextension, PIP and DIP flexion joints; thumb adducted and flexed	MCP joints flexed; PIP and DIP joints extended; thumb in palmar opposition and slight extension	Static splint to hold fingers and joints in functional position, to preserve web spaces
Hip	Flexion, abduction, and external rotation	Neutral alignment, no rotation; hip can be abducted 10 to 15 degrees if burn includes inner thigh to prevent contact with opposite thigh and maceration of burn wound	Wedge, towel, or sheet rolls; plastic splints

Note: MCP = metacarpophalangeal joint; DIP = distal interphalangeal joint; PIP = proximal interphalangeal joint.

TABLE 9-1 (CONTINUED)			
Knee	Flexion	Extension	Before grafting, towel roll under Achilles' tendon; may require plastic, fabric, or KO after grafting; avoid pressure in popliteal fossa or on peroneal nerve at fibular head
Talocrural joint	Plantar flexion	Neutral	Night AFO-SA; check daily for irritation on heels

Orthoses for Walking

One of the best ways to maintain lower-extremity joint mobility, muscle strength, and motor control is to enable the patient to stand and walk as soon as medically feasible. Individuals can begin weight-bearing on a tilt-table. By increasing the amount of time spent in a weight-bearing position and the vertical orientation of the table, the person increases tolerance to the upright posture and improves readiness for ambulation. Splints can be used to stabilize the knees in extension. For patients with plantar flexion contractures, plastic solid ankle-AFOs can be made to accommodate the contracture. This arrangement provides the patient with a base of support suitable for ambulation. For the person with weak dorsiflexor muscles, an AFO with a plastic or metal dorsiflexion assist is useful.

Orthoses for Pediatric Burn Care

Pediatric patients present special challenges to the burn team. Children have thinner, more fragile skin than adults and are likely to sustain more severe injuries. Youngsters often have little insight into cause-and-effect relationships, so they may not understand how they got injured and the rationale for participating in the rehabilitation program. To encourage use, orthoses can be made in the child's favorite color or decorated with decals of the patient's favorite cartoon characters or athletic team logos. Burn rehabilitation may continue for years. Unlike adults, who can usually resume their customary lives on discharge from a burn unit, children are more likely to have to return periodically for scar revisions and new orthoses because growth may foster deformity.[13]

ORTHOSES FOR PATIENTS WITH SOFT TISSUE PROBLEMS ASSOCIATED WITH NEUROMUSCULAR DISORDERS

Management Issues

Patients with myopathies or central or peripheral neuropathies share many problems with those who sustain burns, particularly vulnerability to forming deformities and reduction of functional ability. Consequently, many orthoses designed for burn management can be used for those with neuromuscular disorders.

Orthoses can be a very effective part of a total rehabilitation program for individuals with neuromuscular diseases, which include soft tissue problems. The clinician must perform a comprehensive evaluation, then set individualized treatment goals for the patient. To the degree that orthoses can help achieve long- and short-term goals, they are valuable components of rehabilitation.

Preventing Deformity

Preventing or managing joint contractures necessitates that health professionals emphasize functional activities rather than static positioning. Boys with Duchenne's muscular dystrophy who remained ambulatory had minimal plantar flexion contractures if they wore AFOs at night to control foot and ankle alignment.[14,15] Once they became dependent on wheelchairs, they rapidly formed ankle contractures.[16]

Upper extremity involvement (eg, as seen in arthrogryposis) responds to splints that position the hands, wrists, and elbows. The patient with shoulder girdle and elbow weakness may benefit from orthotic components added to the wheelchair. A lap tray, forearm trough, or sling suspension can maintain good joint alignment as well as enable maximal independent function.[17]

Increasing Range of Motion

Orthoses can be used to increase joint range of motion. They may be part of a postsurgical protocol or be a nonsurgical means to manage soft tissue tightness.

Serial casting is a technique employed to stretch tendons, muscles, and other soft tissues. It involves manually stretching the joint to its maximum length, then applying a plaster cast to hold the body segment in the extended position. After several days or weeks, the cast is removed. Usually, the joint is manually stretched again and a new cast applied. An individualized treatment protocol determines how often the cast is changed and how many times the procedure is repeated. Factors such as age, diagnosis, and presence and severity of increased muscle tone, as well as skin tolerance to casting, determine the treatment protocol.

Alternatives to serial casting are serial static splinting and progressive serial splinting. In the former, splints are reshaped as the range of motion increases; in the latter, orthoses have mechanisms for adjustment. Another option is continuous passive motion applied by a machine, which has a motor that continuously moves a splint on the limb. The machine can be programmed to operate for a specific duration and can be adjusted to move the joint through a predetermined range of motion.

Preventing Pressure Sores

Individuals with considerable musculoskeletal weakness are vulnerable to pressure sores, also known as decubitus ulcers. Bony prominences are especially susceptible to tissue breakdown. Splints, positioning devices, and wheelchair cushions and bolsters can redistribute forces, thereby reducing the risk of sores (Figure 9-5). The devices remove focal points of pressure by redistributing and dissipating weight-bearing forces over a larger surface area. They are most effective when used in conjunction with a comprehensive program that includes repositioning the patient every 2 hours, daily range of motion, stretching, and strengthening exercises.

Promoting Function

Orthoses can help patients with upper-limb weakness resume daily activities. The movement involved in eating, dressing, and similar tasks can help reduce contractures while providing the patient with the

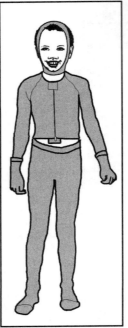

Figure 9-5. Protective orthosis that applies force over a large area of the body.

psychological and physical benefits of self-care. Those who have trunk and lower limb paralysis may wear orthoses to promote ambulation. For example, boys with Duchenne's muscular dystrophy are often fitted with orthoses, whether or not surgery is performed.[18-20] A pair of lightweight polypropylene KAFOs with a solid ankle set in 90 degrees and drop-lock knee joints is sometimes prescribed. The knee lock with pretibial or suprapatellar band, or a knee pad prevents knee flexion contracture. Patients may require a walker, crutches, or canes for walking. An ankle and knee stretching program can also promote function, although its frequency and duration are controversial.[15]

SUMMARY

Orthoses are used temporarily in the management of burns, wounds, and other soft tissue disorders. Orthoses used in burn care include splints, positioning devices, and pressure garments. Burn team members have adopted an approach that permits patients more freedom of movement and less encumbrance with restrictive equipment. Contemporary management fosters healing, which results in pliable tissue, rather than hypertrophic scarring. Patients with soft tissue problems use orthoses to help achieve specific treatment goals: to promote continuing independent ambulation, to prevent deformity, to prevent pressure sores, and to increase range of motion. Static splinting, serial static splinting, progressive serial splinting, and continuous passive motion machines can prevent soft tissue contractures and maintain or increase joint range of motion.

THOUGHT QUESTIONS

1. Explain how a pressure garment helps shape a maturing scar.
2. What are the differences between serial splinting, static splinting, and progressive serial splinting? Explain why you would favor one approach over the other. Describe an ideal candidate for each device.
3. Design a dynamic hand splint to provide traction on the metacarpophalangeal joints while enabling resistive exercise of the finger flexors. Describe all the components of this splint.
4. Design a dynamic splint that will enable a patient to increase range of motion of metacarpophalangeal joints 2 through 5.
5. Describe at least three orthoses that can position a burn patient's neck in extension.
6. Explain why continued ambulation is the best way to prevent plantar flexion contracture in individuals with Duchenne's muscular dystrophy.

REFERENCES

1. Richard R, Staley M, Miller S, Warden G. To splint or not to splint—past philosophy and present practice: part I. *J Burn Care Rehabil.* 1996;17:444-453.
2. Richard R, Staley M, Miller S, Warden G. To splint or not to splint—past philosophy and present practice: part II. *J Burn Care Rehabil.* 1997;18:64-71.
3. Richard R, Staley M, Miller S, Warden G. To splint or not to splint—past philosophy and present practice: part III. *J Burn Care Rehabil.* 1997;18:252-255.
4. Fricke NB, Omnell ML, Dutcher KD, et al. Skeletal and dental disturbances after facial burns and pressure garments. *J Burn Care Rehabil.* 1996;17:338-345.
5. Fricke NB, Omnell ML, Dutcher KA, et al. Skeletal and dental disturbances in children after facial burns and pressure garment use: a 4-year follow-up. *J Burn Care Rehabil.* 1999;20:239-249.
6. Staley MJ, Richard RL. Burns. In: O'Sullivan SB, Schmitz TJ, eds. *Physical Rehabilitation: Assessment and Treatment.* 4th ed. Philadelphia, Pa: FA Davis; 2001:845-872.
7. Ward RS. Pressure therapy for the control of hypertrophic scar formation after burn injury: history and review. *J Burn Care Rehabil.* 1991;12:257-262.
8. Evans EB, Alvarado MI, Ott S, McElroy K. Prevention and treatment of deformity in burn patients. In: Herndon DN, ed. *Total Burn Care.* Philadelphia, Pa: WB Saunders; 1996:443-454.
9. Flynn AE, Gunter LL. Rehabilitation of the burn patient. In: Martyn JAJ, ed. *Acute Management of the Burned Patient.* Philadelphia, Pa: WB Saunders; 1990:320-332.
10. Malick MH. *Manual on Management of the Burn Patient Including Splinting, Molding, and Pressure Techniques.* Pittsburgh, Pa: Harmarville Rehabilitation Center; 1982.
11. Mann R, Yeong EK, Moore M, et al. Do custom-fitted pressure garments provide adequate pressure? *J Burn Care Rehabil.* 1997;18:247-249.
12. Giele H, Liddiard K, Booth K, Wood F. Anatomical variations in pressures generated by pressure garments. *Plast Reconstr Surg.* 1998;101:399-406.
13. Ott S, McElroy K, Alvarado MI, et al. Treating deformities via positioning and splinting, using skeletal suspensions and traction, and with prosthetics and orthotics. In: Herndon DN, ed. *Total Burn Care.* Philadelphia, Pa: WB Saunders; 1996:454-470.
14. Scott OM, Hyde SA, Goddard C, Dubowitz V. Prevention of deformity in Duchenne's muscular dystrophy: a prospective study of passive stretching and splintage. *Physiotherapy.* 1981;67:177-180.
15. Stuberg WA. Muscular dystrophy and spinal muscular dystrophy. In: Campbell SK, ed. *Physical Therapy for Children.* Philadelphia, Pa: WB Saunders; 1995:295-324.
16. McDonald CM. Limb contractures in progressive neuromuscular disease and the role of stretching, orthotics, and surgery. *Phys Med Rehabil Clin N Am.* 1998;9:187-211.
17. Pedretti LW, Zoltan B. *Occupational Therapy: Practice Skills for Physical Dysfunction.* St. Louis, Mo: Mosby-Year Book; 1990:332-344.
18. Siegel IM, Miller JE, Ray RD. Subcutaneous lower limb tenotomy in the treatment of pseudohypertrophic muscular dystrophy. *J Bone Joint Surg [Am].* 1968;50:1437-1443.
19. Heckmatt JZ, Dubowitz V, Hyde SA, et al. Prolongation of walking in Duchenne's muscular dystrophy with lightweight orthoses: review of 57 cases. *Dev Med Child Neurol.* 1995;27:149-154.
20. Shapiro F, Bresnan MJ. Orthopaedic management of childhood neuromuscular disease, part III: disease of muscle. *J Bone Joint Surg [Am].* 1982;64:1102-1107.

CASE STUDIES

For the following cases, select appropriate orthoses, establish long- and short-term treatment goals, and develop a treatment plan.

- RM, a 59-year-old part-time cook, has a 45-year history of alcohol abuse. He sustained circumferential deep partial-thickness and full-thickness burns to both feet, ankles, legs, thighs, and lower torso when he climbed into a scalding bath and fainted. He was found unconscious in the tub by his daughter, who called the paramedics and had him admitted to a burn unit.

- BG, a 38-year-old salesman, sustained full-thickness and deep partial-thickness burns to his face and anterior neck from hydrochloric acid thrown by his angry ex-wife. The plastic surgeon has put skin grafts over the wounds and has requested orthotic management to minimize scarring.

- OC, 18 months old, has spastic cerebral palsy and has just started walking. She walks on her toes. Her physician is considering lengthening the Achilles' tendons surgically to bring her feet plantigrade. When she is in a relaxed position, the physical therapist can obtain 10 degrees of passive dorsiflexion bilaterally after a vigorous stretching program. At the request of her mother and physical therapist, her physician has agreed to a trial program of serial casting or progressive static splinting instead of the surgery.

- GH, a 14-year-old student, was kicked in the head during a football game. He has been in a coma since the injury. The CT scans show severe injury in the thalamus. The nursing staff has requested a consultation for suggestions on positioning.

- JH, a 68-year-old semiprofessional female golfer, had a total knee replacement. One day after surgery, she has active range of motion of 15 to 85 degrees. The surgeon has requested a consultation on orthotic management of this patient.

- MM, 8 years old, has Duchenne's muscular dystrophy. He is still ambulating independently but is developing a severe lumbar lordosis. He walks very slowly and holds onto walls and tables to avoid falling. He has bilateral hyperpronation of his feet and increasing weakness in both quadriceps (3/5). He has difficulty climbing stairs and rising from supine to standing. He has been referred to the orthotic clinic for evaluation.

- PN, a 6-month-old with spastic cerebral palsy and severe mental retardation, is attempting head control and swiping at objects. He was born with bilateral fisted thumbs. His mother noted that he never opens his hands. She wondered if hand splints could help. PN's physician has referred him to the orthotic clinic for an evaluation.

POINT/COUNTERPOINT

KF, a 24-year-old data-entry clerk, sustained deep partial-thickness burns to the right hand, wrist, and forearm when she tried to light her gas oven after the pilot light had extinguished. She is right-handed and lives alone.

| JOAN SAYS | JAN SAYS |

Orthotic Prescription

Because this is a circumferential burn, a custom-molded plastic wrist-hand stabilizer with finger separators should be placed over the volar surface to prevent flexion contractures. The stabilizer should extend to the antecubital fossa. The orthosis is molded to maintain the interphalangeal joints extended, the metacarpophalangeal joints flexed, the transverse palmar arch curved, the thumb abducted and opposed, the wrist slightly extended with neutral deviation, and the forearm partially pronated. The stabilizers are secured with broad dorsal straps. Interdigital separators prevent adduction contractures.

An elastic gauntlet glove should be worn over the stabilizer to minimize hypertrophic scarring. A single-strap sling will reduce edema.

I agree. I am particularly concerned about preventing unsightly hypertrophic scarring on this young woman's hand and forearm.

Long-Term Goals

Maintain full mobility of all fingers, as well as the wrist and forearm. Restore normal skin flexibility and appearance. She cannot afford to take much time off from work, so she needs to accomplish all daily, household, and vocational activities independently. This may involve learning to use her left hand for tasks that are ordinarily bimanual.

A major concern is preventing infection in such an extensive burn. I want to reduce her pain to a manageable level and help her to be independent in skin care as well as in functional activities.

Short-Term Goals

Maintain full active range of motion of interphalangeal and metacarpophalangeal joints, wrist, and forearm, as well as thumb opposition. Minimize hypertrophic scarring and skin reddening. Mobility should be achieved within 3 weeks. Skin restoration should occur within 6 weeks. She should be able to accomplish daily and basic household activities independently within 1 week.

Reduce pain by at least two levels on the visual analog scale. Teach her skin care to prevent infection. Suggest ways in which she can perform daily activities, using assistive devices as needed. She should be independent in range-of-motion exercises and donning and doffing orthoses.

| JOAN SAYS | JAN SAYS |

Treatment Plan

Instruct the patient in one-handed dressing, grooming, feeding, and writing activities with her left hand. Plan a bathing program so that she can maintain shoulder support while keeping the injured hand and forearm dry. As soon as the splint and glove are removed, institute active-assisted exercises in which she uses her left hand to mobilize the right hand and forearm. Guide the patient in hand and forearm massage with graduated pressure as the skin heals.

Instruct her in independent donning and doffing of her orthoses. Teach her how to perform range-of-motion exercises with her left hand. I agree that she also needs instruction in ways of facilitating daily and vocational activities with the left hand. This may involve helping her to select clothing styles and fastenings that are easy to manage. Instruct her in wound care and skin care.

Chapter 10

Goal Setting and Treatment Planning

*"Walk on, walk on, with hope in your heart
And you'll never walk alone."*
Oscar Hammerstein, *Carousel*

After the clinician has determined that orthotic management is indicated, the next step is to develop appropriate long-term goals, short-term goals, and a treatment plan with the patient.[1-3] Setting goals for orthotic management encompasses three broad categories: preventing impairments, reducing functional limitations, and minimizing disability. The American Physical Therapy Association defines these terms in the *Guide to Physical Therapist Practice*.[4]

LONG-TERM GOALS

Long-term goals refer to restoring the individual to his or her desired role in society. According to the *Guide to Physical Therapist Practice*, an impairment is the "loss or abnormality of a physiological, psychological, or anatomical structure or function."[4] Using this definition, appropriate long-term goals for orthotic management include reducing pain, preventing soft tissue contractures, promoting normal muscle strength, restoring full joint range of motion, and averting musculoskeletal deformity.[5] Table 10-1 lists long-term goals for orthotic management to prevent impairments.

Functional limitations are restrictions to a person's ability to perform a given duty or activity in the customary manner. Orthoses designed to minimize functional limitations can be used to improve dynamic equilibrium, assist balance, and promote a better performance of activities of daily living. Examples of long-term goals that improve dynamic equilibrium include independence in walking on level surfaces, transferring from bed to a wheelchair with contact guarding, and rolling from side-to-side in bed with minimal assistance. Orthoses that assist balance can aid a person while sitting or standing. To promote better performance of daily activities, orthoses have been designed to enable independence in feeding, dressing, and personal hygiene. Long-term goals for orthoses designed to minimize functional limitations are provided in Table 10-2.

The third category of orthotic goal-setting concerns minimizing disability. In this context, "disability" describes a personal status that prevents a person from acting in an appropriate social role in a given social setting within a specific physical environment.[6] A long-term goal for orthotic management of a high school football player with an unstable knee would be to minimize further injury to the knee

---

TABLE 10-1

Long-Term Goals:
Orthotic Management for Preventing Impairments

- Prevent deformities
- Prevent or reduce edema
- Maintain or improve joint mobility
- Prevent hypermobility
- Increase joint stability
- Achieve optimal joint alignment
- Distribute pressure tolerably
- Prevent hypertrophic scarring
- Increase strength
- Minimize or decrease pain

TABLE 10-2

Long-Term Goals:
Orthotic Management for Functional Limitations

- Achieve the maximal level of independent ambulation
- Transfer independently from all surfaces
- Achieve independence in bed mobility
- Perform all feeding, food preparation, and clean-up activities independently
- Accomplish all personal hygiene and grooming activities independently
- Dress and undress independently
- Perform all household cleaning and routine maintenance activities independently
- Do all garden and lawn care activities independently
- Operate a motor vehicle independently
- Perform the usual tasks of the patient's occupation independently
- Engage in the usual leisure time activities independently

---

during the playing season. More examples of long-term goals for orthotic management to minimize functional limitations appear in Table 10-3.

SHORT-TERM GOALS

Short-term goals are derived from long-term goals. Each short-term goal must be observable, measurable, and have a designated duration. For example, a patient who has a foot drop resulting from peroneal neuropathy has difficulty walking 5 meters without tripping. The person is in relatively good health and is very motivated to regain the ability to walk normally. A long-term goal might be independent ambulation on level surfaces and stairs using an AFO-PLS. When the individual first puts on the orthosis, he has poor dynamic balance and limited endurance. A short-term goal might be "Patient will be able to ambulate safely on a level surface with an AFO-PLS for 35 meters twice daily with contact guarding in 2 weeks." Practice writing short-term goals is provided at the end of this chapter.

TABLE 10-3

Long-Term Goals:
Orthotic Management for Disability

- Resume the role of husband or wife
- Function in the role of parent
- Resume the role of high school student and varsity athlete
- Participate with one's peers in preschool activities

TREATMENT PLANNING

After long- and short-term goals, the next step in rehabilitation is developing a treatment plan. The plan should enable the patient to achieve the short-term goals within the stated duration and the long-term goals by time of discharge. Training in donning and doffing the orthosis and education about proper care for the appliance and the underlying skin are always part of treatment planning, which involves an orthosis.

The clinician should explain to the patient that an accommodation period is necessary so that the skin and underlying soft tissues can adapt to the new appliance. The length of the accommodation period depends on the extent of bracing and the person's physical condition. Someone needing a KAFO who has poor skin integrity, considerable weakness, and multiple contractures will take longer to accommodate than a strong, healthy athlete who is receiving foot orthoses.

Initially, after the orthosis has been evaluated and delivery is accepted, the patient should wear the orthosis for no longer than 2 hours at a time. It should be removed and the skin inspected. Any red areas should be reexamined after 5 to 10 minutes to see if the skin returns to its normal color. Persistent redness, blisters, or wounds require that the patient discontinue wearing the orthosis and contact the clinician who dispensed it as soon as possible.[7] If the person tolerates wearing the orthosis on a limited basis, the wearing time can then be increased gradually. Each time the period is extended, the individual should inspect the skin upon doffing the orthosis. In this manner, tolerance to wearing the orthosis can be increased until it can be worn safely full-time.

Orthoses for the lower limb interact with the shoe and the walking surface. Patients should be taught to manage uneven terrain, steps, slopes, and unstable surfaces such as sand, gravel, and ice. Those fitted with AFO-SAs should be aware that walking on irregular or resilient surfaces can result in inadver-

tent knee flexion. Strategies such as ascending ramps sideways with the foot perpendicular to the slope or using a zigzag "tacking" approach can accomplish the task. Individuals without major cognitive impairments should be encouraged to develop their own techniques for coping with environmental problems, so they can feel in control while wearing the appliance. While the patient experiments with different approaches to a given task, the clinician should guard the person against injury and provide feedback as to the merits of each experiment. Clinicians should become familiar with the various places that their patients frequent, then discuss with the patient the challenges that each place may pose. For especially risky situations, the clinician and patient might visit the place to try the orthosis. Alternatively, reproducing the hazards in the clinic will let the patient attempt various solutions to the problem.

For patients with severe cognitive impairments, the clinician should analyze the task, divide the task into its components, and then train the patient in each subtask. For example, the clinician may begin by helping the person identify a surface as being either level or irregular. Next, one chooses a specific strategy for the client and trains the person in that strategy. Simple sayings can reinforce training, helping the person remember the technique. For example, for negotiating stairs: "Up with the good [foot] and down with the bad [foot]." When walking on slippery surfaces: "When you slide, feet walk wide." This should remind the client to widen the walking base.

CRITERIA FOR DISCHARGE

Patients may be discharged from treatment when the long-term goals have been achieved or when the clinician determines that the original goals are unrealistic. In the latter instance, one should revise the goals; discharge is appropriate when the patient achieves the revised goals.

Some people object to wearing an orthosis. They may find it unattractive, heavy, or difficult to use. Those who refuse to use their orthoses may be discharged from treatment because they are no longer deriving benefit from orthotic intervention. Hopefully, good communication between the patient and all members of the treatment team will result in a discharge that is mutually agreeable.

CARE OF ORTHOSES

A structured program of orthotic care[8-9] should be part of every treatment plan in order to enable the orthosis to function properly for the anticipated duration of use. Orthoses should be laid in extended alignment on a table or on the floor when not worn.

Components

Shoes

- Air dry the shoes nightly; ideally, alternate shoes from day to day to allow for full airing, assuming the shoes can be separated from the rest of the orthosis
- Use shoe trees to maintain the original shape of the shoes
- Shake the shoe before donning it to dislodge any debris
- Keep heels and soles in good repair
- Inspect linings to make certain they are intact, not worn or torn; if so, replace the shoe
- Check the interior of the shoe for any protruding nails from the sole
- If the shoe is riveted to a stirrup, examine the rivets to make certain that none have separated; if rivets are loose, return the orthosis to the orthotist for repair
- Protect the shoes from snow, mud, and torrential rain; if shoes become wet, insert shoe trees or stuff them with newspaper and allow them to dry away from direct heat

Plastic Shells

- Wipe with a cloth moistened with a diluted solution of mild soap and water
- Do not soak the orthosis in cold or hot water
- Do not dry the orthosis with a hair dryer or other heater
- Avoid contact with heat, such as leaving it in a car parked in the sun
- Check for surface blemishes, which may indicate exposure to heat

- Maintain constant body weight and control any edema to avoid edge pressure
- In a child's orthosis, check the fit of shells every 3 months to make certain that their edges do not indent the soft tissue. If a shell has become too small, return to the orthotist with the child and the orthosis so that it can be enlarged

Metal Joints

- Keep joint surfaces clean; inspect and remove debris with a cotton swab or fine wire, such as a hairpin
- Once a week, lubricate joints with a drop of machine oil, taking care not to let oil drip on leather or fabric components
- Check the locking mechanism to make certain it functions smoothly; if not, return the orthosis to the orthotist

Metal Uprights

- Inspect the orthosis weekly to check for loose or missing screws or bolts and replace them if necessary
- In a child's orthosis, check every 3 months to make certain that the orthosis still fits properly

Metal Bands

- In a child's orthosis, check the fit of bands every 3 months to make certain that the edges of the bands do not indent the soft tissue. If a band has become too small, return to the orthotist with the child and the orthosis so that it can be enlarged

Materials

Leather

- Interior surface of bands is usually upholstered with horsehide, which can be wiped with a cloth moistened with a diluted solution of mild soap and water
- Exterior surfaces of bands are usually covered with cowhide; a cloth moistened with saddle soap will remove surface stains
- Other leather parts are usually made of cowhide, which can be cleaned with saddle soap

Fabric

- Wear clean fabric between the orthosis and the skin; for lower-limb orthoses, cotton hose is suitable because the fabric absorbs perspiration. Nylon hose reduces friction. Hose should be slightly higher than the top of the orthosis. Upper-limb orthoses should be worn over tubular cotton or synthetic stockinette. Sacral, lumbosacral, and thoracolumbosacral orthoses should be worn over a cotton t-shirt. Cervical orthoses should be worn over stockinette.

- Synthetic fabrics, if detachable, can be washed in a washing machine on gentle cycle
- Other fabrics can be spot cleaned

Accessories

Buckles

- Inspect buckles to make certain they are in good repair

Laces

- Check laces, particularly at places in which the laces contact rigid surfaces
- Replace laces every 6 months to avoid unanticipated breakage

Straps

- Clean hook-and-pile straps with a toothbrush moistened with diluted soapy water to enable the closure to seal properly; debris from the environment and clothing tends to accumulate in surfaces of the straps
- Inspect leather and fabric straps, particularly at places in which the straps contact rigid surfaces, and replace as necessary

Wires

- Protect wires from moisture
- Avoid exerting excessive traction on wires, particularly when the orthosis is worn while the wearer transfers from one seat to another

Batteries

- Recharge batteries nightly
- Obtain a second set of batteries to be used while the primary set is being recharged or if the original batteries need replacement
- Check the batteries with a voltage meter every 6 months to determine whether they function optimally; if they do not, replace the batteries

SUMMARY

When orthotic management is indicated, the clinician should develop long- and short-term goals and a treatment plan. Setting goals encompasses preventing impairments, reducing functional limitations, and minimizing disability. Short-term goals are derived from specific long-term goals and must be observable, measurable, and have a stated duration. Treatment plans enable patients to achieve their goals. Plans should include training regarding donning, doffing, care of the orthosis, and care of the skin. An accommodation period enables the patient to get accustomed to wearing the appliance. Clinicians should acquaint clients wearing lower extremity orthoses to maneuver over hazards in the environment and let the individuals develop strategies for coping with the problems. The clinician should guard the patient from injury and provide feedback during the strategy sessions. Those who have cognitive deficiencies benefit when the clinician provides a strategy and trains the person in the specific approach. Patients may be discharged from treatment when the long-term goals have been met or when the clinician determines that the individual will derive no benefit from additional intervention. Care of the orthosis involves regular inspection and attention to the condition of the components, materials, and accessories.

THOUGHT QUESTIONS

1. Differentiate between long- and short-term goals.
2. Outline an accommodation period for a patient with spinal cord injury at T8 who has been provided with THKAFOs.
3. How can the clinician instruct the patient with cognitive impairment in the safe use of an AFO-PLS?
4. Susan, a 12-year-old with scoliosis, refuses to wear her orthosis. Suggest several techniques that may help her to comply with the treatment plan.

REFERENCES

1. Coulehan JL, Block MR. *The Medical Interview: A Primer for Students of the Art.* 2nd ed. Philadelphia, Pa: FA Davis; 1992.
2. Kleinman A. *Patients and Healers in the Context of Culture: An Exploration of the Borderland Between Anthropological Medicine and Psychiatry.* Berkeley, Calif: University of California Press; 1980.
3. Parry K. Culture and personal meanings. *PT Magazine.* 1994;2:39-45.

4. American Physical Therapy Association. *Guide to Physical Therapist Practice.* Alexandria, Va: American Physical Therapy Association; 1999.

5. McCollough NC. Biomechanical analysis systems for orthotic prescription. In: American Academy of Orthopaedic Surgeons. *Atlas of Orthotics.* 2nd ed. St. Louis, Mo: CV Mosby; 1985:34-75.

6. Verbrugge L, Jette A. The disablement process. *Soc Sci Med.* 1994;38:1-4.

7. Marshall AT. *Care & Use Guide: Plastic Ankle-Foot Orthosis.* Alexandria, Va: American Academy of Orthotists and Prosthetists; 1986.

8. Edelstein JE. Orthotic assessment and management. In: O'Sullivan SB, Schmitz TJ, ed. *Physical Rehabilitation: Assessment and Treatment.* 4th ed. Philadelphia, Pa: FA Davis; 2001:1025-1060.

9. Redford JB. Principles of orthotic devices. In: Redford JB, ed. *Orthotics Etcetera.* 3rd ed. Baltimore, Md: Williams & Wilkins; 1986:1-21.

RECOMMENDED READING

Lower Limb Orthotics. New York, NY: New York University; 1986.

Establish long- and short-term goals, and develop a treatment plan for the following cases.

- AB is a 66-year-old retired house painter who has a left peroneal neuropathy from years of exposure to lead-based paints. He has non-insulin-dependent diabetes and cannot feel light touch or distinguish sharp and smooth stimuli on the soles of either foot. He had cataracts removed from both eyes and now wears thick eyeglasses. He received an AFO-PLS that has been evaluated and accepted as satisfactory. Mr. B's wife accompanies him to therapy sessions. They boast that they are celebrating 40 years of wedded bliss. Mrs. B is concerned about her husband's health and wants to do "whatever it takes" to get him back on his feet and healthy again.

- FV is a 72-year-old widow who has left-sided spastic hemiplegia. Her left foot is held in 10 degrees of plantar flexion and her left knee buckles then snaps into hyperextension when she steps on the limb. She has a 1-inch subluxation of her left glenohumeral joint; her left hand is fisted and nonfunctional. She has left-sided homonymous hemianopsia, left-sided neglect, and dressing apraxia. She also has slurred speech and tends to drool from the left side of her mouth. The orthotic clinic prescribed a hemispiral AFO, a wrist-hand stabilizer, and a shoulder sling.

- DT is a 36-year-old telephone repairman who sustained second- and third-degree burns to his face, hands, and forearms when charcoal ignited while he was trying to get a barbecue started in preparation for his son's birthday party. Splints were made for both hands and forearms; a mask was molded for his face. Mr. T is concerned about whether he will be able to return to work.

- MC is a 2-year-old girl with spina bifida who has no sensation or motor control below L4. She is developmentally delayed. She is now starting to pull herself to the standing position and cruise along a sofa. She has been fitted with bilateral AFO-SAs and has been referred to your clinic for therapy.

- RA is a 12-year-old student with idiopathic scoliosis. She recently had a growth spurt, resulting in an increase in the curvature. She dislikes the body jacket because it is hot, bulky, and conspicuous. Her physician warned that if the curvature cannot be controlled with the brace, she will have to stabilize the spine surgically.

- FN is a 47-year-old accountant who sustained amputation of three fingers of his left hand when his daughter accidentally slammed the car door on his hand. The fingers have been surgically reattached. He has been fitted with a wrist-hand stabilizer and a finger flexor orthosis.

Professional Organizations

American Board for Certification in Orthotics and Prosthetics, Inc.
330 John Carlyle Street
Alexandria, VA 22314
703-836-7114

American Congress of Rehabilitation Medicine
5987 East 71st Street
Suite 111
Indianapolis, IN 46620
317-915-2250

American Academy of Orthopaedic Surgeons American Orthopedic Association
6300 North River Road
Rosemont, IL 60018
847-318-7330

American Orthotic and Prosthetic Association
330 John Carlyle Street
Alexandria, VA 22314
703-836-7116

American Occupational Therapy Association
4720 Montgomery Lane
PO Box 31220
Bethesda, MD 20824-1220
301-652-2682

American Physical Therapy Association
1111 North Fairfax Street
Alexandria, VA 22314-1488
703-706-3395

Association of Children's Prosthetic-Orthotic Clinics
6300 North River Road
Suite 727
Rosemont, IL 60018-4226
847-698-1637

Board for Orthotist/Prosthetist Certification
506 West Fayette Street
Suite 200
Baltimore, MD 21201
410-539-3910

Interdisciplinary Society for the Advancement of Rehabilitative and Assistive Technology
1700 North Moore Street
Suite 1340
Arlington, VA 22209
703-524-6686

International Society for Prosthetics and Orthotics
Borgervaenget 5
2100 Copenhagen Ø
Denmark
45-3920 7260

Pedorthic Footwear Association
7150 Columbia Gateway Drive
Suite G
Columbia, MD 21046
800-673-8447

Sources for Orthoses, Materials, and Components

Acor Orthopaedic, Inc
18530 South Miles Parkway
Cleveland, OH 44128
800-237-2267

AliMed
297 High Street
Dedham, MA 02026
800-225-2610

Apex Foot Health Industries, Inc
414 Alfred Avenue
Teaneck, NJ 07666
201-833-2700

Atlanta International
1979 Parker Court
Suite E
Stone Mountain, GA 30087
800-543-7660

Ballert International, Inc
3645 Woodhead Drive
Northbrook, IL 60062
800-345-3456

Becker Orthopedic
635 Executive Drive
Troy, MI 48083-4576
248-588-7480

Bio-Concepts, Inc
2424 East University Drive
Phoenix, AZ 85034
800-421-5647

Birkenstock
8171 Redwood Boulevard
Novato, CA 94945
800-949-7321

Bledsoe Brace Systems
2601 Pinewood Drive
Grand Prairie, TX 75051
800-527-3666

Boston Brace International, Inc
20 Ledin Drive
Avon, MA 02322
800-262-2235

Camp Healthcare
2690 Cumberland Parkway
Suite 222
Atlanta, GA 30339
770-333-9700

Cascade Orthopedic Supply
1000 Fortress
Suite 900
Chico, CA 95973
800-888-0865

Cascade Prosthetics and Orthotics, Inc
1360 Sunset Avenue
Ferndale, WA 98248
800-848-7332

Center for Orthotics Design, Inc
561 Division Street
PO Box 37
Cambell, CA 95008
800-346-4746

DOBI Symplex
Division of Seattle Orthopaedic Group
26296 Twelve Trees Lane NW B-1
Poulsbo, WA 98370
800-248-6463

Fillauer, Inc
PO Box 5189
2710 Amnicola Highway
Chattanooga, TN 37406
800-251-6398

Generation II USA
11818 North Creek Parkway North #102
Bothell, WA 98011
425-486-9057

Hapad, Inc
5301 Enterprise Boulevard
Bethel Park, PA 15102
800-544-2723

Innovation Sports
19762 Pauling
Foothill Ranch, CA 92610
800-222-4284

IPOS North America
2045 Niagara Falls Boulevard
Suite 8
Niagara Falls, NY 14304
800-626-2612

Jobst
653 Miami Street
Toledo, OH 43605
800-537-1063

Langer Group, Inc
450 Commack Road
Deer Park, NY 11729
800-233-2687

Lenox Hill Division of Seattle Orthopaedic Group
26296 Twelve Trees Lane NW B-1
Poulsbo, WA 98370
800-248-6463

Liberating Technologies, Inc
71 Frankland Road
Hopkinton, MA 01748
800-437-0024

PW Minor & Son
3 Treadeasy Avenue
Batavia, NY 14020
716-343-1500

North Coast Medical
18305 Sutter Boulevard
Morgan Hill, CA 95037
800-821-9319

Oregon Orthotic System
2280 Three Lakes Road SE
Albany, OR 97321
800-866-7522

Ortho-Craft, Inc
1 Action Boulevard
Londonderry, NH 03053
800-436-7846

Orthomedics
180 North San Gabriel Boulevard
Pasadena, CA 91107
626-796-8733

Orthomerica Products, Inc
PO Box 2927
Newport Beach, CA 92659
800-637-4500

Orthotic Technical Supply
735 North Fork Road
Barnardsville, NC 28709
800-221-4769

Otto Bock Orthopedic Industry, Inc
Circle Star Warehouse
14630 28th Avenue, North
Plymouth, MN 55447
800-328-4058

Palumbo Orthopaedics
8206 Leesburg Pike
Suite 405
Vienna, VA 22182
800-292-7223

Pel Supply
4666 Manufacturing Road
Cleveland, OH 44135
800-321-1264

Restorative Care of America, Inc
11236 47th Street North
Clearwater, FL 34022
800-627-1595

Rieken's Orthotic Laboratory
5115 Oak Grove Road
Evansville, IN 47715
800-331-8040

Sammons Preston
4 Sammons Court
Bolingbrook, IL 60440
800-323-5547

Scott Orthotic Lab
1831 East Mulberry Street
Fort Collins, CO 80524
970-484-5017

Silipos, Inc
7049 Williams Road
Niagara Falls, NY 14304
716-283-0700

Smith & Nephew Rolyan, Inc
1 Quality Drive
PO Box 1005
Germantown, WI 53022
800-558-8633

Smithers Oasis
919 Marvin Avenue
Kent, OH 44240
800-321-8286

Spinal Technology, Inc
191 Mid Tech Drive
South Yarmouth, MA 02763
800-253-7868

Townsend Design
4615 Shepard Street
Bakersfield, CA 93313
800-432-3466

Ultraflex Systems
534 Trestle Place
Trestle Bridge Business Center
Downingtown, PA 19335
800-220-6670

United States Manufacturing
180 North San Gabriel Boulevard
Pasadena, CA 91107
800-228-5448

Viscolas
8801 Consolidated Drive
Soddy Daisy, TN 37379
800-548-2694

Websites for Orthotic Materials, Products, and Other Resources

Websites are subject to change. Please check the URL or use a search engine if webpages do not load.

3-Point Products
http://www.3pointproducts.com
Elbow and shoulder orthoses, finger and thumb orthoses, foam plastic, hand and wrist orthoses.

About Face
http://www.aboutfaceinternational.org
About Face is an international organization that provides information and emotional support to individuals with facial differences and their families.

Action Products, Inc
http://www.actionproducts.com
Orthosis liners.

Aircast Inc
http://www.aircast.com/
Ankle-foot orthoses.

Alberta Burn Rehabilitation Society
http://www.burnrehab.com/
The mission of the ABRS is to assist those who have suffered through the trauma of a serious burn injury and to prevent serious burn injuries through education.

AliMed, Inc
http://www.alimed.com/
Orthoses and orthotic fabrication materials for ankle-foot orthoses, elbow and shoulder orthoses, finger and thumb orthoses, foam plastic, hand and wrist orthoses, head and neck orthoses, hook-and-pile fasteners, knee orthoses, orthosis liners, and trunk and cervical orthoses.

American Burn Association
http://www.ameriburn.org/
Information and interactive communication on burn care and related research, teaching, rehabilitation, and prevention issues.

Becker Orthopedic
http://www.beckerorthopedic.com/catalog.htm
Orthoses and components.

Best Priced Products, Inc
http://www.best-priced-products.com
Ankle-foot orthoses, hook-and-pile fasteners.

Bio-Concepts, Inc
http://www.bio-con.com/index.html
Custom- and ready-made pressure garments for compression therapy in burn scar management.

Bio Med Sciences, Inc
http://www.silon.com/
Silicone plastic for face splints.

Bledsoe Brace Systems
http://www.bledsoebrace.com/
Knee-ankle-foot orthoses.

Boston Brace
http://www.bostonbrace.com/
Trunk and lower-limb orthoses.

Brace Archive
http://www.geocities.com/HotSprings/3825/
cti.htm
Knee orthoses, halo traction, scoliosis orthoses, links to other sites, and clubs.

BSM-JOBST
http://www.jobst-usa.com
Gradient compression stockings and bandages.

The Burn Foundation
http://www.aarbf.org/
The Burn Foundation works in partnership with firefighters, educators, and burn care professionals to develop programs and services.

Burn Institute
http://www.burninstitute.org/
The Burn Institute is dedicated to reducing the number of burn injuries and deaths in San Diego and Imperial counties in California.

Burn Support Group Database
http://www.burnsupportgroupsdatabase.com/
Worldwide support groups listed in eight languages including burns, disfigurement, cleft-lip.

Burn Survivors Dictionary
http://www.members.tripod.com/~vudue/dict.html
Glossary of terms pertaining to burns, burn survivors, and their families.

Burn Survivors Online
http://www.burnsurvivorsonline.com
Peer support for patients with burns.

Burn Survivors Ribbon Campaign
http://www.members.tripod.com/~vudue/ribbon.html
Burn survivors' support online.

Camp Healthcare
http://www.camphealthcare.com/ortho.html
Orthoses and components.

Castroom
http://castroom.com/
Website devoted to plaster casts.

Changing Faces
http://www.changingfaces.co.uk/
Facial disfigurement and its social and emotional consequences; started by a man with facial burns.

Chattanooga Group, Inc
http://www.chattgroup.com
Ankle-foot orthoses, elbow and shoulder orthoses, finger and thumb orthoses, knee orthoses, orthosis liners.

CMO, Inc
http://www.cmo-inc.com
Elbow and shoulder orthoses, hand and wrist orthoses, knee orthoses, trunk orthoses.

Connecticut Coalition For Organ and Tissue Donation
http://ctorganandtissuedonation.org/
Information on tissue donation.

Corflex, Inc
http://www.corflex.com
Ankle-foot orthoses, elbow and shoulder orthoses, finger and thumb orthoses, head and neck orthoses, hook-and-pile fasteners, knee orthoses, orthosis liners, and thermoplastics.

DeRoyal
http://www.deroyal.com
Thermoplastics, ankle-foot orthoses, elbow and shoulder orthoses, finger and thumb orthoses, foam plastics, hand and wrist orthoses, trunk orthoses, hook-and-pile fasteners, orthosis liners.

Doctor's Guide—Global Education
http://www.pslgroup.com/dg/3e19e.htm
University of Chicago Burn Center replaces hand-drawn charts of a patient's wounds with a morphable three-dimensional computer body image.

DonJoy Orthopedics
http://www.donjoy.com/
Knee orthoses.

Dynatronics
http://www.dynatronics.com/
Ankle-foot orthoses, hook-and-pile fasteners, thermoplastics.

Eastern Orthopaedics
http://www.eortho.com/
Orthoses for the major joints and trunk.

Empi
http://www.empi.com
Elbow and shoulder orthoses, knee orthoses.

Essex Orthopaedics
http://www.essexorthopaedics.co.uk/page5.htm
Upper limb, lower limb, and spinal orthoses.

Fillauer, Inc
http://www.fillauer.com
Ankle-foot orthoses, elbow and shoulder orthoses, hand and wrist orthoses, head and neck orthoses, hook-and-pile fasteners, knee orthoses, orthosis liners, trunk orthoses.

FlagHouse
http://www.flaghouse.com
Ankle-foot orthoses, elbow and shoulder orthoses, finger and thumb orthoses, hook-and-pile fasteners, knee orthoses.

FLA Orthopedics, Inc
http://www.flaorthopedics.com
Ankle-foot orthoses, elbow and shoulder orthoses, finger and thumb orthoses, knee orthoses.

FootSmart
http://www.footsmart.com/
Ankle-foot orthoses, podiatric products.

Foundation for Burned Children
http://www.fondtomafound.org/
This Canadian bilingual (French and English) site provides access to articles, organizations, news about burns and burn victims, computer downloads, games, and support groups. It has webpages from Disney.com that should provide hours of entertainment for children of all ages.

Generation II USA, Inc
http://www.gen2.com
Ankle-foot orthoses, knee orthoses, orthosis liners.

Georgia Firefighters Burn Foundation
http://www.gfbf.org/
Founded in 1982 by a group of Atlanta-area firefighters, the foundation's mission is to educate the public in burn awareness and prevention, to support medical facilities in the care of burns in Georgia, and to assist burn survivors in their recovery.

Hanger Orthopedic
http://www.hanger.com
Ankle-foot orthoses, elbow and shoulder orthoses, finger and thumb orthoses, foam plastic, hand and wrist orthoses, head and neck orthoses, hook-and-pile fasteners, knee orthoses, orthosis liners, trunk orthoses.

High Desert Riders, Inc.
http://www.highdesertriders.net
High Desert Riders, Inc promotes self-development in individuals, youth groups, community and service organizations, and businesses.

Human Interface Technology Lab—Washington University
http://www.hitl.washington.edu/projects/burn/
Advanced treatments for burn survivors.

IMAK Products Corp
http://www.imakproducts.com
Elbow and shoulder orthoses, finger and thumb orthoses.

InnovationSports
http://www.isports.com/
Sporty knee braces for children, athletes, and people with osteoarthritis.

International Society for Prosthetics and Orthotics
http://www.i-s-p-o.org/
Interdisciplinary organization.

Joint Active Systems, Inc.
http://www.jointactivesystems.com/
Ankle-foot orthoses, elbow and shoulder orthoses, hand and wrist orthoses, knee orthoses.

The Joint-Jack Co
http://www.jointjackcompany.com
Wrist-hand orthoses.

KC Regional Firefighters' Burn Foundation
http://www.kcburn.org/
A nonprofit organization dedicated to public safety education, community development programs involving fire safety, promotion of the fire services to the public, prevention of burn injuries, and the recovery and rehabilitation of burn survivors and their families, and the families of deceased or injured firefighters.

Lenjoy Medical Engineering, Inc
http://www.comfysplints.com
Ankle-foot orthoses, hand and wrist orthoses, knee orthoses, orthosis liners.

Loyola University Health System
http://www.lumc.edu/
Research investigating problems in post-burn immunosuppression, wound healing, and nutritional support.

MA Rallis Corp
http://www.rallis.com
Ankle-foot orthoses, elbow and shoulder orthoses, hook-and-pile fasteners, knee orthoses.

Mayo Clinic Resource Site
http://www.mayo.edu/staff/plastic/Cosmetic/CSOLMain.html
Cosmetic surgery information.

MEDdirect
http://www.shopmeddirect.com
Ankle-foot orthoses, elbow and shoulder orthoses, wrist-hand orthoses, knee orthoses.

Mueller Sports Medicine
http://www.muellersportsmed.com/splints.htm
Air splints for fractures.

National Center for the Dissemination of Disability Research
http://www.ncddr.org/rr/burn/burn1.html
Contains a QuickTime movie on hypertrophic scarring.

National Institute of General Medical Sciences
http://www.nih.gov/nigms/news/facts/
Fact sheets on trauma and burn injury statistics, research, and resources.

Orthomerica Products, Inc
http://www.orthomerica.com
Ankle-foot orthoses, elbow and shoulder orthoses, hand and wrist-hand orthoses, head and neck orthoses, knee orthoses, orthosis liners, trunk orthoses.

Orthotics and Prosthetics Digital Technologies, Inc
http://www.oandp.com/
Orthotic components.

Otto Bock Health Care
info@ottobockus.com
Ankle-foot orthoses, elbow and shoulder orthoses, hand orthoses, knee orthoses, thermoplastics.

Patient Care Services—UC Davis Medical Center
http://www.pcs.ucdmc.ucdavis.edu/ptcare/burn.htm
The Burn Recovery Support Group is a monthly peer-support meeting.

The Phoenix Fire Department
http://www.ci.phoenix.az.us/FIRE/burns.html
The Phoenix Fire Department provides basic information about burns, with instructions for classifying burns, determining their severity, and treating them.

Prosthetics and Orthotics Information Online
http://www.pando.com
Canadian prosthetics and orthotics resource.

Restorative Care of America, Inc
http://www.rcai.com
Ankle-foot orthoses, elbow and shoulder orthoses, wrist-hand orthoses, knee orthoses, trunk orthoses.

Road Runner Sports
http://www.roadrunnersports.com/
Shoe critic section for reviews of brands of shoes and models; "medical tent" section for advice on Achilles' tendonitis, plantar fasciitis, runner's knee (chondromalacia), shin splints, iliotibial band syndrome, sciatica, side stitch; and bicycle accessories section for knee orthoses.

Sammons Preston
http://www.sammonspreston.com
Ankle-foot orthoses, elbow and shoulder orthoses, foam plastic, hand and wrist-hand orthoses, head and neck orthoses, hook-and-pile fasteners, knee orthoses, thermoplastics, trunk orthoses.

Pearson and Pearson—A Professional Corp
http://www.pearsonandpearson-law.com/
Information for burn survivors.

Shriners Hospitals
http://www.shrinershq.org/
Shriners Hospitals for Children, a network of 22 hospitals, provide expert, no-cost orthopaedic and burn care to children under 18.

Smith & Nephew Rehabilitation
http://www.smith-nephew.com
Ankle-foot orthoses, elbow and shoulder orthoses, hand and wrist-hand orthoses, head and neck orthoses, hook-and-pile fasteners, knee orthoses, orthosis liners, thermoplastics, trunk orthoses.

Sports Medical Rehab
http://www.smrproducts.com
Ankle-foot orthoses.

SWB Elbow Brace, Ltd
http://www.swbelbow.com
Elbow and shoulder orthoses.

Swede-O, Inc
http://www.swedeo.com
Ankle-foot orthoses.

Symmetric Designs, Ltd
http://www.symmetric-designs.com
Elbow and shoulder orthoses, knee orthoses, head and neck orthoses.

TCP, Inc
http://www.antiscald.com/facts.htm
Information on scald burns.

Tecfen Corp
http://tecfen.com/emergency/junkin/safin.html
Air splints for fractures.

Townsend Design
http://www.townsenddesign.com/postop.html
Knee orthoses.

Trauma.org—Burns and Cold Injuries
http://www.trauma.org/eates/ectc/ectc-burn.html
Information on burns and cold injuries.

Ultraflex Systems, Inc
http://www.ultraflexsystems.com
Ankle-foot orthoses, hand and wrist-hand orthoses, knee orthoses.

United States Manufacturing Company
http://www.usmc.com
Ankle-foot orthoses, elbow and shoulder orthoses, hand and wrist-hand orthoses, head and neck orthoses, hook-and-pile fasteners, knee orthoses, orthosis liners, trunk orthoses.

University of Rochester Medical Center—Burn Trauma Unit
http://www.urmc.rochester.edu/strong/burn/
Burn-trauma unit at Strong Memorial Hospital.

University of Washington Burn Center—The Fires of Pain
http://www.washington.edu/alumni/columns/dec96/fires1.html
Use of drugs, hypnosis, and virtual reality for burn pain.

University of Western Australia—Second Skin PTY, Ltd
http://www.cs.uwa.edu.au/~bruce/burns/commsite/burnsskn.html
Pressure garment manufacturer.

Vanserve Site—Burn Survivor Resource on the Web
http://www.vanserve.org/vanservehome.htm
Burn information resource.

WFR Corp
http://www.reveals.com
Thermoplastics.

Index

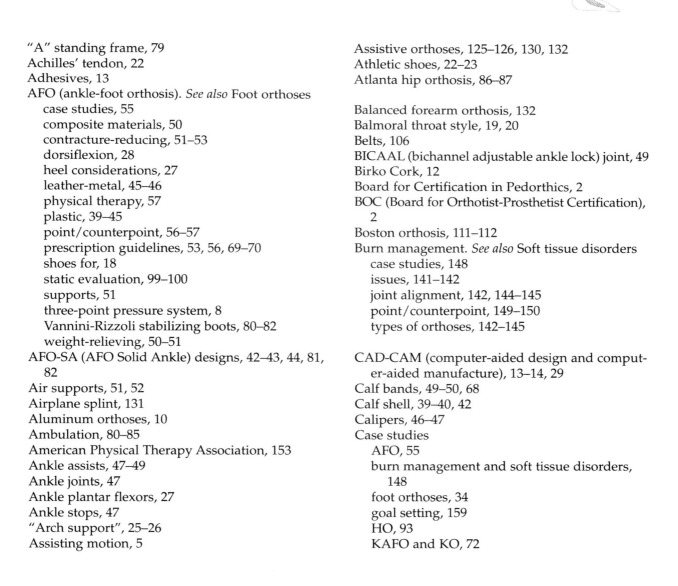

BUILD *Your Library*

This book and many others on numerous different topics are available from SLACK Incorporated. For further information or a copy of our latest catalog, contact us at:

Professional Book Division
SLACK Incorporated
6900 Grove Road
Thorofare, NJ 08086 USA
Telephone: 1-856-848-1000
1-800-257-8290
Fax: 1-856-853-5991
E-mail: orders@slackinc.com
www.slackbooks.com

We accept most major credit cards and checks or money orders in US dollars drawn on a US bank. Most orders are shipped within 72 hours.

Contact us for information on recent releases, forthcoming titles, and bestsellers. If you have a comment about this title or see a need for a new book, direct your correspondence to the Editorial Director at the above address.

Thank you for your interest and we hope you found this work beneficial.